Volume 1

INTRODUCTION TO A
SOCIAL WORKER

INTRODUCTION TO A
SOCIAL WORKER

THE NATIONAL INSTITUTE FOR
SOCIAL WORK TRAINING

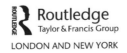

Routledge
Taylor & Francis Group

LONDON AND NEW YORK

First published in 1964 by George Allen & Unwin Ltd.

This edition first published in 2022
by Routledge
2 Park Square, Milton Park, Abingdon, Oxon OX14 4RN

and by Routledge
605 Third Avenue, New York, NY 10158

Routledge is an imprint of the Taylor & Francis Group, an informa business

British Library Cataloguing in Publication Data
A catalogue record for this book is available from the British Library

ISBN: 978-1-03-203381-5 (Set)
ISBN: 978-1-00-321681-0 (Set) (ebk)
ISBN: 978-1-03-205960-0 (Volume 1) (hbk)
ISBN: 978-1-03-205965-5 (Volume 1) (pbk)
ISBN: 978-1-00-320006-2 (Volume 1) (ebk)

DOI: 10.4324/9781003200062

Publisher's Note
The publisher has gone to great lengths to ensure the quality of this reprint but points out that some imperfections in the original copies may be apparent.

Disclaimer
The publisher has made every effort to trace copyright holders and would welcome correspondence from those they have been unable to trace.

INTRODUCTION TO A
SOCIAL WORKER

produced by

THE NATIONAL INSTITUTE
FOR SOCIAL WORK TRAINING

London

GEORGE ALLEN & UNWIN LTD

RUSKIN HOUSE MUSEUM STREET

FIRST PUBLISHED IN 1964
SECOND IMPRESSION 1967

PRINTED IN GREAT BRITAIN
in 10 on 11 point Times Roman type
BY C. TINLING AND CO. LTD.,
PRESCOT

PREFACE

This book is an introduction to social casework, that is to say, it is concerned with social work with individuals and families. It does not set out to discuss the methods used in social work with groups or with communities. The purpose is to present in simple terms a few of the important aims and concepts of social casework and to illustrate some of its methods.

The book is written primarily for students who are starting their training in social work; we hope that it will prove useful to other students in social studies courses. It is written also for those in the community who meet people in trouble and who may not know the help that social work can offer, those who may consider entering the profession, and others who just wonder what it is all about.

In the preparation of this book the National Institute has been assisted by a generous and imaginative grant from the Institute of Social Welfare. This grant enabled us to have the help of Miss Florence Mitchell for six months. During this time she carried out the preparatory task of consulting tutors in social work about the kind of book needed for beginning students, she also prepared much of the text of this book, incorporating case material she had collected over a period of time, as well as the records in chapters III, IV and V which are contributed by other social workers.

Miss Mitchell, now tutor in charge of the course in general social work at Croydon Technical College, brought to this task an intimate knowledge of social work, experience as a teacher and the ability to elicit interest and help for this co-operative enterprise. The book was thus shaped in the course of discussion with practitioners and tutors and with help from Dr E. L. Younghusband and Miss K. M. Lewis, Advisers in Social Work Training at the National Institute. We are grateful to all those whose help has made this publication possible.

R. Huws Jones

CONTENTS

CHAPTER I

PEOPLE WHO NEED
SOCIAL WORK HELP

THE term social worker means different things to different people. For the purpose of this book a social worker may be described as one who helps people and families who have social problems or who are under some heavy stress which they cannot cope with by themselves. It is necessary to make clear what kind of problems, what sort of people have them, what kind of stress social workers are concerned with and how they can help.

Life in a highly organized society is complicated. Most people manage somehow, but some may need help to surmount difficulties and if appropriate help is not available at the right time family breakdown can occur. This applies specially to people who are inadequately equipped financially, physically or mentally or in other ways to meet the struggle of life, or who lack the strong backing of family and friends to see them through in time of trouble. It is necessary to consider different kinds of people and the stresses they may experience before discussing the part played by social workers in helping them.

Most people at some time or other have had to face problems that disrupt their lives—illness, bereavement, financial loss, a severe shock of some kind or just the accumulation of small troubles which, coming on top of the ordinary demands of life, can seem almost unbearable. The most efficient man or woman can be temporarily disabled by a sudden crisis and it would be a very unusual person who did not at some time or other experience difficulties that made his life miserable until the right solution was found.

Because most people want to be independent, they will try to work out their problems by themselves if they can. Some will struggle on indefinitely rather than ask for help, and most of these will come to terms with the difficulty in some way, though it may be with harmful results to themselves and others. Many, however, when their own efforts fail, will seek help from a friend or from their family doctor, their minister or priest, someone whom they trust and to whom they can pour out their troubles in the hope of getting wise counsel. Their counsellor may be able to help them or may advise them to go to a social worker, or they may come direct to a social work agency.

If their problem is simply failure to understand the intricacies of applying for sickness benefit for example, or not knowing where to obtain a passport, or whether the landlord has the right to put up the rent, all they need is straightforward and accurate answers to questions. They can do the rest themselves. The Citizens' Advice Bureaux exist to deal with problems of this sort, but such questions may also be brought to a variety of people who may either answer them themselves, or refer the enquirer to the appropriate agency to give the help he needs.

Sometimes what is needed is material help, residential care, an allowance from the National Assistance Board, an appliance for a physically handicapped person. At other times, to provide the material remedy alone will only touch the fringe of the difficulty or provide only temporary relief. Consider the case of a mother who comes to a social agency saying that she has been advised to go into hospital for an operation but has no one with whom she can leave her children. A practical suggestion may be that the children should be received into the care of the local authority while their mother is in hospital, but this may meet with little response from the client.[1] She needs first to talk over her

---

[1] The word client is generally used to describe the person who comes to a social worker asking for help. It is a term that many social workers dislike but no one has yet been able to think of a better one. In this book for the sake of clarity the client will usually be referred to as 'him' and the social worker as 'her'. In reality many social workers are men and many clients are women.

anxiety about her illness and pending operation, her distress at leaving her children, and her fears about the sort of place they are going to and whether they will be properly looked after. Only when the worker has helped her to come to terms with these anxieties can she accept the practical measures which will meet her need. Moreover, the father's and the children's feelings must also be considered. The social worker must have the knowledge and imagination to understand what disturbances in family life mean in a child's world. In the case of a very young child separation from home might be too disturbing, and alternative plans, such as bringing in a home help or temporary housekeeper may be considered. The worker must weigh up all the factors in the case, the emotional ones as well as the practical, for to social workers 'feelings are facts' and must not be ignored.

The amount of strain which any individual can tolerate without breaking varies very much between one person and another. It depends on temperament and past experience but everyone has some breaking point and when difficulties pile up one upon another all of us reach a point when we feel we can no longer cope without some help from outside. For example, finding somewhere to live is, in present circumstances, extremely difficult for many people. Young couples with small children and a modest wage packet are dependant on a lucky find, or on taking their turn on the local authority's housing list. The waiting period can impose strains that would be unbearable even to a well established family; living with relatives, living in cramped conditions, and attempting to pay hire purchase deposits on furniture while paying a high rent, are common situations. Some people can tolerate these things in the hope of having a home of their own one day; others, less poised, find the strains more than they can bear.

An example of this is the case of a young medical student. He was living on a meagre grant from public funds. He was married and had a delicate wife and a baby. The only accommodation they could get in reach of his work was a furnished flat at five guineas a week which they could afford only by cutting down on food and other necessities. He would not let his child go short so he managed on as little as possible himself. His wife had been advised to go into hospital for treatment and they did not know what to do about the baby while she was away. He did not want her put into a children's home as he had unhappy memories of having been in one when he was a child, but his in-laws refused to take the child because they had strongly disapproved of the marriage. He said that his wife was 'wonderful', but she 'suffered from nerves' and 'things were getting her down'. Even the landlady was being difficult. Under the strain of all these worries he found himself unable to concentrate on his work, and feared he might fail in his examinations, yet it was imperative that he became qualified as soon as possible— he did not know how they were going to get through the next three years anyway. It was a vicious circle from which he could see no escape. Clearly there was a danger that this otherwise happy marriage might break under the strain that was being imposed upon it. In this case the practical problems gave rise to the emotional ones but it could just as well have been the other way round. A social worker might help them to get additional financial help or cheaper accommodation. She might also help them to look again at the estrangement with the wife's parents. The fact these were now grandparents and had also probably got over the first shock of their daughter's marriage might make them glad of a good reason to let down the barriers they had built up.

Strained relationships between individuals or groups of individuals can also set up conflicts which result in a social breakdown. A family may be in danger of disruption through conflicts between husband and wife or parent and children. Conflict with in-laws can lead to marriage difficulties and conflict between partners can wreck a business. More often than not the person who is suffering under emotional stress carries his unhappiness and bad temper out of the house with him and it affects other areas of his life. The man who has quarrelled with his wife at breakfast is likely to arrive at work edgy and ready to row with the foreman. He may lose his job if this happens too often. The wife who feels her husband does not appreciate her may cheer herself up by spending the rent money on a new perm (a nice way of annoying her husband). The child who has slept badly, because his parents were quarrelling all night in the next room, goes to school tired and has difficulty in concentrating on his lessons. If this goes on he may fail in his examination and miss the chance of the higher education his parents had set their heart on. One thing leads to another. One isolated incident does not constitute a social problem, but an accumulation of incidents may well build up into something that seriously affects the life, not only of the person concerned, but of many other people directly or indirectly connected with him. We are all members of society and the private troubles of the individual are ultimately the concern of all.

In some cases the root of the problem lies in the client's personality. Some people's make-up is such that they are always in trouble. Although skilled workers, they can never keep a job; although their income is adequate they are always in debt; although they have many acquaintances they have no real friends. When the difficulties of a person's temperament combine with circumstances that seem overwhelming to him, he usually needs someone right outside his family circle to help him to see his problem in perspective and to sort things out. The task needs great skill, for he is generally blind to the part his own character plays in bringing about his misfortunes, and blames them all on other people or circumstances beyond his control. Before he can be helped to put things right he must be helped to gain insight into what has gone wrong.

So far we have been considering problems that stem from lack of knowledge, from lack of material necessities, from problems of stress through sudden catastrophe, from difficulties piling up or from problems of relationship and of personality. We must now consider the problems of the person who suddenly suffers a calamity which perhaps completely disrupts his life. Maybe he was previously a capable, self-reliant man; now, through no fault of his own, he finds himself dependent on others and forced to change his whole way of life. Perhaps he was a skilled craftsman but his accident has rendered him unfit for his work: he may be offered an unskilled job suitable to his condition, but until he has become reconciled to the fact that he can never hope to regain his former skill or return to his highly paid, responsible post, he is likely to resist all efforts to help him. 'Help' for him consists of standing by him in the distress of disablement and encouraging him gradually to see that physical injury does not imply a loss of personal worth. The failure to provide his family with their former income does not imply that he has ceased to be a responsible husband and father. Only when he has been helped to realize that he is still a person of value to his family and to society is he likely to be able to think about alternative ways of earning a living. Such was the situation of Mr Thomas, a skilled metal worker, earning good money and with prospects of becoming head of his department. A road accident left him with little use in one leg and no hope of continuing his trade. Because of his excellent work record the firm offered him a job in the office, responsible, but to him inferior. As he discussed it with the firm's personnel manager, Mr Thomas was on the point of tears and banged his caliper on the floor in his frustration at his disablement. He said he was no good to anyone in this state; he didn't want the job—it was just paper stuff—but he would have to take it because no one else would have him; he had let down the wife and kids; they had hoped to get a new house, but they'd never manage it now. Instead of slapping Mr Thomas on the back saying that it was not really so bad, and urging him to cheer up, the personnel manager said he could understand Mr Thomas feeling like that; he thought it was very hard to know you had a skill and could never use it again, but he wondered if it really made Mr Thomas such a different person. He knew the directors had been very keen to keep him because of his expert knowledge of metals and he thought he was still very important to his family. Mr Thomas was sceptical, but he came back a week later, saying he had been talking it over with the wife. She told him she was so thankful he hadn't been killed she didn't care what they had to go without so long as he was still around. He had never thought he meant so much to the old girl. As a matter of fact, things weren't so bad: they would have to wait longer for the house, but they could still have it before the kids grew up, and he had decided to take over the job of honorary secretary of the tenants' association. They had been on at him for a bit but he had refused because he thought it was only because they were sorry for him.

When a person has been worrying over some difficulty and turning it over in his mind until he is quite confused, it is a great help to him to be able to talk it over with some understanding person who will respect his confidence. The obvious person to confide in would seem to be a close friend or a member of his family who knows him and his circumstances. Often a 'listening ear' is all that is needed. Putting the problem in words helps to clarify it and releases tension so that things fall into perspective and the sufferer himself may find his own solution or may find that the other person's point of view has thrown new light on the problem. Many people solve their problems with the aid of friends or family; but this kind of help is not always sufficient. Friends and relatives can sometimes be very helpful and sometimes the reverse. It is often difficult to admit failure to one's own family; the attitudes and advice of different members of the family may conflict; they may even be part of the cause of the trouble; in any case relatives are liable to be so full of sympathy and protectiveness that they are incapable of seeing the full picture. Friends too may become involved and indignant on one's behalf, or scornful of one's inability to cope. Advice from friends is rarely helpful because a friend tends to see your problem in *his* way and fails to see what is bothering *you*. Untrained helpers can rarely resist the temptation to give advice, which often confuses more than it clarifies the issue.

B

Someone who is threatened with a lawsuit, if he is wise, will consult a good lawyer, or someone seriously ill will consult a doctor in preference to trying home remedies; so the man or woman who is suffering from the kind of problem we have been discussing is well advised to seek the help of someone professionally qualified to help him in these matters. But even as a doctor cannot always cure his patient, so there is no magic by which social workers can find an infallible remedy for social ills. All they do is to try to the best of their ability to help the client to put right what is wrong with his life. In the last analysis it is how the client himself uses the help that counts.

Professional social workers are not immune from human weaknesses but at least they come to the situation free from direct emotional involvement and are trained to look at the situation objectively; therefore they are more likely to see it as a whole. They try to see a situation through the eyes of a person whose problem it is and to understand what it means to him. It is not easy to get inside another person and understand his way of thinking, feeling, acting and responding to a situation, yet it is just these personal characteristics which may have caused or aggravated the problem.

Knowledge of ways in which people normally behave and react to others, and how this normal behaviour is altered in times of stress, helps a trained social worker to understand what is happening to the individual concerned and to other people involved with him in the problem. By training and experience the social worker learns to recognize some of the patterns of behaviour common to people in trouble, and some of the ways in which they defend themselves when they feel threatened by other people or by circumstances. Some will fight, some will run away, some will become very worried, while others deny that there is anything wrong.

This knowledge of human behaviour provides a background to the social worker's understanding of the problem, but, as no two people react in exactly the same way to any situation, the social worker must try to understand the character of the client, how his past experiences have combined to influence his reaction to his present circumstances, and what strength he has in his character to meet and overcome his difficulty. She will try to understand how the problem looks to him, and what solution, if any, he has thought of. If this is realistic she will support him in carrying it out, but if not, she will try to help him to see the situation more clearly and aid him to the best of her ability to find a satisfactory solution. Although she will sometimes give practical or material aid where she feels this would help to meet the total problem, her main work will be through what is called the casework relationship which will be discussed more fully in the next chapter.

The purpose of the method is to help people in trouble to remain or to become independent and self-respecting citizens. This method is not simple. It has to be learned and practised. It stems from social work experience and draws heavily on knowledge from the social sciences and psychology which throw light on people's needs and behaviour. This knowledge must be combined with skill in specific ways of helping, and with compassion for people in distress within a framework of ethical values.

The ethical values which underlie casework, are:

(a) to respect the client;
(b) to accept him for himself;
(c) not to condemn him;
(d) to uphold his right to self determination; and
(e) to respect his confidence.

These all grow out of the ideals embodied in the democratic principles of our western way of life, with its emphasis on the value of each unique individual. Some find expression in our social legislation, and in the concept of the welfare state. These ideals are familiar, though we tend to pay lip service to them rather than to live up to them, especially when it comes to the misfits in our own society. Social work, in common with some other professions, is a conscious and systematic attempt to translate these values into terms of professional practice and to see how they apply to the needs of individuals in distress, particularly those whose troubles are caused by their inability to fit into the society around them.

Respect for the individual in his right as a human being is grounded in certain religious and humanist views about the nature of man. This principle has always been as fundamental to social work as the Hippocratic Oath is to medicine. Lesser principles follow from it.

Social workers strive to accept the individual as he is whether or not he measures up to their idea of what he should be. They must so far as possible feel goodwill towards him, desire his well-being and show this by the warmth of their response to him. To maintain this feeling towards all clients is not easy, for social workers are, of course, human and cannot like everyone equally. Some clients may be rather unpleasant people and may do things of which no one could possibly approve. Yet if they feel they have to act a part in order to win goodwill how can they possibly tell social workers the truth about themselves or their problems? The more that is learnt of the difficulties which have driven them to behave in the way they do the easier it often becomes to accept them, but initially acceptance means an attitude of receptiveness, a willingness to see things from the client's point of view. It means looking for the best in people and recognizing the bad without either condemning or condoning it.

This immediately leads to the problem of non-condemning attitudes. If social workers do not condemn are they not in danger of condoning? When they accept the individual who is breaking the law or the moral standards of society it does not mean that they approve his actions or pretend to do so—it may even on occasion be appropriate to express disapproval—but acceptance means that social workers do not condemn him as a person because of his acts, or punish him by becoming indifferent about him. It is the condemnation and indifference which destroys the relationship and it is the worker's real feeling, whether positive or negative which gets across to the client. Words of acceptance mean nothing if they are not sincere. The problem of maintaining a non-condemning attitude is illustrated in the case of Mrs Bristoe in Chapter V where the worker refrains from direct criticism and shows understanding of the client's difficulties but at the same time makes her face up to the reality of the situation in which she finds herself as a result of her misconduct. Social work does not stop at accepting people as they are. This is the first step towards helping them to become better—to use their own strengths.

The individual's right of self-determination stems from the democratic principle of freedom of choice, with its attendant right of non-comformity. It is a sign of maturity to want to make one's own decisions and chose one's way of life, but these rights must be set in the context of the individual's obligations as a member of society. The individual has the right to make his own decisions, but sometimes he is too young, too unrealistic or too sick to be able to do so; sometimes he is too immature or too lacking in confidence to want to do so; and sometimes he is too anti-social to be allowed to do so. The social worker must sometimes take some measure of control, guide the client, and set limits to his behaviour. In most socially irresponsible people there is some degree of immaturity which tends to make them dependent on the social worker. The importance of bearing in mind the principle of the client's right to self-determination comes from the fact that there is a subtle temptation in most of us to rule the lives of other people if we get the chance, there is also satisfaction in feeling that the client needs us. He may need others to take charge temporarily, but the social worker will always strive to restore his independence as soon as possible. For a strong-minded and capable worker, who sees the client struggling with something which could easily be done for him, to forbear and leave him the satisfaction of accomplishing it himself calls for real professional self-discipline. Yet to build up confidence and responsible behaviour is an essential aim of social work.

Confidentiality would seem to be the easiest principle to adopt since we can readily understand that the client does not want to have his private affairs bandied about. This is why the principle of confidentiality is beginning to become a common practice. But because it means weighing up one thing against another its application sometimes presents considerable difficulties. There are problems connected with communicating confidential information to colleagues or other agencies, and as to whether the client's permission should always be asked before divulging confidential information or whether there are occasions when this is not appropriate. The practice will also vary to some extent between different agencies. However, social workers should keep the principle of confidentiality constantly in mind because this shows respect for aspects of his life which the client regards as private.

The principles we have been discussing relate to the worker's attitude to the client: their meaning must be clarified in each particular situation. Often social workers are faced with moral problems which will require a reassessment of their own values or their ethics in a professional role. Recognition of long-treasured prejudices and a deepened self-awareness may be painful. But social workers who do not know themselves and their motives have little hope of knowing their clients, who like them are individuals with strengths and weaknesses There are no such beings as perfect social workers, there are only those who try their best with whatever gifts have been granted to them to help other people. Natural gifts are not evenly distributed but whatever they may be at the beginning they can be strengthened by training, by greater professional maturity, and by making use of the knowledge and experience of others. This all broadens understanding and deepens insight into the client's needs. It can also increase self-awareness and the professional self-discipline and integrity whereby social workers learn to face their own less attractive characteristics while they are working with the client and to use their good qualities to the best advantage to help other people These demands in varying forms are made on members of all professions.

For centuries people inspired by a sense of vocation and guided largely by intuition have worked to alleviate the hardships suffered by the casualties and outcasts of society. What then is new about casework? Perhaps partly the fact that it is a systematic attempt to gather together the experience of social workers in the past and present, to use available scientific knowledge, and to evolve methods and principles of practice. These methods will be illustrated later when we are considering the casework relationship itself. As the social workers of the future contribute in their turn to the common pool, the reservoir of knowledge will widen and deepen. We are only just beginning the task and have a long way to go before we have anything like the wealth of knowledge and skill which the medical profession, for example, can bring to bear on the problems of physical illness, but at least we have made a start.

CHAPTER II

THE METHODS OF SOCIAL WORK

THE relationship established between the social worker and the client is the heart of casework. It is unlike yet like the other relationships of everyday life. It is different from the relationship between parent and child, with its strong biological ties; it is different from friendship, which arises out of mutual liking and shared interests and which demands give and take; it is very different from an acquaintanceship with neighbours based on geographical proximity, or with a landlord, bank manager, grocer or postman. Perhaps its nearest parallel is the relationship between doctor and patient, which comes into being because of the patient's illness and ceases when he gets better again. Even here there is a difference, for the patient relies primarily on the doctor to diagnose his symptoms and suggest treatment, but the caseworker and client must work together throughout on the difficult task of understanding and finding a solution to the client's problem. To this joint enterprise the client brings not only his problem but himself; his character, his past and present difficulties, his hopes and fears for the future, his weaknesses and his potentialities. And the caseworker brings her willingness to help, her knowledge and her skill.

The caseworker relationship is thus a professional one existing for the benefit of the client not the caseworker and centred on the problem with which he comes to the agency. It may be quite a strong relationship because of the client's need and the emotions which this rouses both in him and in the social worker, but once the problem is solved the relationship is no longer necessary and can be terminated.

The casework relationship exists for a purpose related to the particular client's need. The danger of failing to remember this is illustrated by the cautionary tale about a woman who had been visiting a social work agency for some years. When her regular worker left she was transferred to a new member of staff. On reading the file the new worker was unsure of the purpose of the interviews, the supervisor could not recall what it was about, and the director of the agency, on being consulted, suggested that the client should be asked. The client was deeply affronted. She said: 'First time I came because my pension hadn't come through; since then I've come because I thought the young lady liked to talk. She always seemed pleased to see me.' This is an extreme example, but it serves as a warning, for it is easy to allow a professional relationship to slip into a social one without realizing what is happening. The client comes with a series of day-to-day problems about which she seeks the case worker's advice and the latter is beguiled into wrestling with these problems without realizing that the client only comes to the office because she enjoys having a nice little chat. To avoid this the case worker must frequently review the situation, reminding herself of the original purpose of the relationship and noting what progress has been made.

When the client is a person who experiences difficulty in his contacts with other people and particularly when this difficulty is combined with emotional immaturity, the development of a good relationship, in which much is given and little is demanded, can provide the sheltered environment necessary for growth and change. There is a natural tendency in all living things to strive towards wholeness and normality. As the doctor uses his skill to aid the recuperative powers of the body, so the caseworker uses hers to support and strengthen the client's desire to put right whatever is wrong with his personal or social adjustment. But if the client really lacks the will to change little or nothing can be achieved.

In the normal development of the personality in childhood the natural processes of growth are stimulated, supported and encouraged by parental love. In the immature adult this normal development has been stunted by adverse circumstances in his past life but the processes continue to some extent if sufficient support and encouragement is provided to stimulate the client's will to grow up. This is not easy but it can be done where the worker's acceptance of, and concern for, the client provides the motive power which sets the process moving.

The foundations of the casework relationship are laid at the first interview between the client and the social worker. This may take place in the client's home or the social worker's office; in court, in a children's home, or in a hospital ward. The client is usually a person in distress and if the social worker shows an obvious desire to help, the client will generally respond. Sometimes this concern is expressed in practical ways, perhaps by visiting the client in hospital or prison, or by helping him with things he finds difficult like filling in forms or making appointments. One social worker used to make a point of writing to patients who were about to undergo a frightening experience, timing it so that the letter arrived on the morning of the ordeal. It is surprising how much comfort can be given by such small acts of consideration. When professional workers in any field do something over and above what can reasonably be expected of them people feel that they really care about them.

Of course much casework consists of clarifying the client's problem by discussion but there is more to the relationship than a verbal exchange of views. There is the subtle influence of one personality on another. This is hard to define. An example which is familiar to everyone is the way in which a child will imitate the gestures, likes and dislikes of an adult he admires. In the same way a social worker who has a good relationship with a young person may achieve more because of this unconscious identification than would ever be achieved through direct admonition. Again we all know people whom it is good to be with when we are feeling low—in many cases it is not primarily what they say but what they are that makes us feel better.

A casework interview is both free-flowing, yet structured and purposeful. The client who comes to a social agency for the first time is likely to feel anxious, to be uncertain whether he has done the right thing. Perhaps he has been trying for a long time to summon up sufficient courage for this visit: he may be reluctant to discuss his problems with a stranger and ashamed of his inability to cope with them. It is important at the outset that the social worker welcomes him and expresses willingness to help, for if he were to be asked too abruptly why he had come, he might take this as a rebuff.

Having welcomed him, the social worker invites him to speak about his problem and leaves him to do this in his own way, for she is concerned not only with the facts he has to tell her but also with the way in which they appear to him. If the tale is very confused she may ask a few questions to help her to understand it, but she will leave most of the talking to him. Talking freely releases some of the client's initial anxiety and makes it easier for him to get down to the problem. This means that the social worker must know how to listen. Listening is indeed a vital part of casework. It will be discussed more fully later in this chapter.

While he is talking and the social worker is listening, she will also be assessing whether this client has needs with which the particular agency is competent to deal. If not, she will suggest to the client that she should refer him elsewhere, for he may not wish to discuss private and painful subjects with her and then have to do it all over again somewhere else. If the problem as it begins to emerge seems to be something with which she can help, she will consider whether there is need for any immediate action or whether she can allow herself time for proper study and assessment of the situation. If there are other people concerned whom she ought to see—for instance some other member of the family, or the family doctor—she will ask the client's permission before doing so.

Assuming that she has decided that this is a case which will require further work, what information will she need in the first or first few interviews? If it is a new problem she needs to know what the client has done already. If it is a long standing one she needs to know how the client coped with it in the past and what has made it seem intolerable now. That is to say, whether his usual way of dealing with it has broken down or whether a new form of stress has aggravated the whole situation so that he now feels it is beyond his control. She attempts to understand the nature and extent of the problem and sometimes to help the client to a clearer understanding of it too. At the same time she tries to assess what resources he has for meeting it or facing its implications. Can he find his own solution with some support? Or must she temporarily take over control of the situation until the client has recovered sufficiently to make his own decisions once more? She will also try to discover whether he has any friends or family who can give support, for it is generally better to get help from home or neighbour-hood than to rely on support from outside. She will not be able to help the client to plan for the future until she has understood the nature of the problem as it affects him and his family. To take immediate action is therefore rarely desirable though circumstances sometimes make it unavoid-able. Time spent in careful systematic study of the situation and of the degree of stress it is causing is necessary to a proper understanding of the problem, the client's capacity to meet it, and the kind of help he will need to do so.

The following simple story illustrates how easily a well-meaning worker could have done the wrong thing if she had given the help asked for without waiting to find out if it would meet the real need.

Mrs Townley was a widow living on National Assistance who telephoned to a casework agency during the week before Christmas asking for money to buy presents for the children. The worker, feeling miserable at having to refuse the re-quest, explained that her organization had no funds and went on to sympathize with Mrs Townley about the worry of being short of money at such a time. After some minutes conversation Mrs Townley said: 'You can't imagine what a relief it's been to have a talk about it. It's not really the presents for the kids, I know my mother will help about them; it's just that it all piled up at that moment and I had no one to tell about it. I should have hated you if you'd offered money.'

While the worker is assessing the client, the client is also assessing the worker—deciding whether this is someone whom he can trust and who is competent to help him. A satisfactory assessment begins a relationship in which the worker and client are already engaged in the task of clarifying the relevant issues. The process of feeling different will often begin before all the facts have been assembled or a plan made. This is because the establishment of the relationship in itself does something to alter the situation in so far as the client begins to experience a measure of confidence and hope.

In first and subsequent interviews the client and social worker sort out what are the most urgent aspects of the problem and look for ways of meeting the difficulties. These may include practical or financial help or referral to other agencies such as a hospital or child guidance clinic. Plans are agreed and the client returns or is visited as necessary to discuss progress and difficulties. There will be both progress and set-backs, but if the client has begun to experience some possibility of change in the situation he usually accepts the social worker's support in his efforts. All her endeavours will be directed towards building up his self-respect and his ability to cope with his own life successfully through a better understanding of himself in relation to his difficulties. This cannot always be achieved, particularly when the client is an immature and child-like person who needs a great deal of support, but it is generally possible to improve his situation even if it cannot be completely cured. When difficulties are, as far as possible, overcome, the reason for the social work service is ended. Many clients, however, will return from time to time for help with setbacks or further problems.

These are some of the ways in which a social worker listens to the client and uses the casework relationship. It is necessary to look a little more closely at what listening means, for there is more than one way of listening. We may hear what is said and yet fail to grasp what the client is trying to convey to us. Human beings communicate in various ways: by words, by gesture, by attitude, by tone of voice, by what is left unsaid, said with great emphasis or said in reverse, for example, 'Of course I'm very *fond* of her but . . .' Clients may also reveal their feelings by their actions, for instance by failing to keep an appointment at which a painful topic is to be discussed, or by arriving late when they are cross with the worker. Of course, though, it is also possible to have simple reasons for being late. By listening to the emotional undertones, the social worker can often understand what is really troubling the client and so be able to help him put into words something he wants to say but is too shy or ashamed to bring out. This can be helpful to both parties. As one social worker put it, 'You must listen to the words and the music.'

Listening to the client's troubles can in itself be helpful, as in the case of Mrs Townley, or there may be a much more profound problem to be discussed and worked through, as with Mr Foster whose case is discussed later. There may be need for practical assistance in an emergency, as with Mrs Bristoe (Chapter V) or for prolonged support, as with Mr Upton (Chapter IV). Sometimes practical, material or financial aid may be necessary and helpful as part of the total plan, but it should not be given as a quick way of trying to help an importunate client when the social worker is too busy to give him proper time and attention. Such help may relieve the symptoms but rarely gets to the root of the problem. The client's feeling about financial assistance is also important. To some people the gift of money when they are in need comes as a welcome present, but to others it seems shameful; as though the giving were a sign of contempt and the taking a sign of failure. In such cases the social worker must consider carefully whether the real need for money outweighs the harm that will be done to the client's self-respect. These feelings about money are illustrated in the case of Mrs Townley, and in those of Mrs Bristoe and Mr Upton to be discussed later.

An important part of listening is quickly recognizing the significance of what is said. Often a casual remark made by the client will give the social worker an opportunity to open up a new aspect of the problem as yet unexplored. For instance the client may refer to a photo on the mantelpiece mentioning that it was her son as a baby, the other lad in the picture, she says, was the boy who was killed. Genuine interest shown by the social worker enables her to talk about the past when her children were young, her difficulties at that time, her distress and depression when her eldest son was killed in a motor accident, the effect this had on other members of the family, and so on—the whole family back ground emerges naturally.

It is not enough to listen, the social worker must also respond appropriately to what the client has to say. This response may be in words or it may be implicit in her actions or her attitude. If it is sincere it will be conveyed to the client, even an inarticulate noise or a gesture suggesting sympathy, understanding or encouragement may be enough. The client needs some indication that the social worker is trying to understand the situation and his part in it. It is not helpful to argue with a client, to talk him down, to offer unwanted advice or to take the problem out of his hands if he can possibly manage it himself.

Failure to listen can result in failure to give help appropriately as in the case of Mr Foster who called at a welfare organization asking for ways of raising funds for his fare to Canada. He mentioned casually that he and his wife were not getting on very well but that she might join him later. His plan seemed reasonable, so the social worker made the necessary enquiries and had the information ready for him when he returned next week. He replied that he had now decided to go to Australia and gave more good reasons. The social worker listened carefully to this change of plan, then remarked that he didn't seem very certain where he wanted to go and she wondered if he really wanted to go anywhere.

At this Mr Foster burst out with the impassioned reply: 'No, I thought you would realize I felt desperate, but you seemed to think it was easy to go to Canada, so I made it as far as I could. But I can't get away from myself and unless I change, my wife won't stay with me. I couldn't just say that to you until I knew what you were like.'

In this case the client seems to have wanted the social worker to help him bring out his difficulty. Yet had she done so too soon, before he 'knew what she was like' he might have denied that he had a marriage problem at all. In these matters timing and tact are all important. The social worker must feel her way, keeping in step with the client. She must try to perceive what is of immediate concern to him and deal with that, while she herself bears in mind the wider issues. Except in dire necessity, the problem that the client brings out initially may not be what is really worrying him. He needs to know the social worker before he trusts her. Sometimes the problem which is troubling the client does not seem to the social worker to be the root of the matter and she is tempted to probe deeper. But here she must be careful not to go too far ahead of the client's understanding. If she asks questions or makes comments that seem to him irrelevant he will be irritated and their good relationship may suffer.

The client's real need may be hidden alike from himself and from the social worker until it becomes apparent after prolonged discussion. This was shown by a client who was seen regularly for six weeks by a social worker at the request of the housing manager. The family was in arrears with the rent but the housing manager was loath to evict them because he felt sure there was some good reason. Each week the wife came to the social work agency and poured out her fury at her husband for not taking a lead in coping with their troubles. The social worker kept bringing the discussion back to the rent arrears and became increasingly anxious because, although the client replied politely, no money was paid off. By the sixth week the worker feared she would have to admit failure. She thought things sounded better at home but still no rent was being paid. Then, just as the client was leaving, she stopped and said: 'D'you know I've suddenly realized I wasn't paying the rent because I was so mad with my husband! We're getting on better now. I'll call at the office and pay it off on my way home.'

Many different kinds of people come to the social worker with their troubles. She has to deal with enquiries, requests for advice, people with marriage problems, problems about children, problems about housing, money, neighbours' quarrels and with multiple problems which often need much sorting out. These external difficulties are inextricably mixed with the client's emotional problems, how he feels about what is happening to him now and what has happened to him in the past; and sometimes difficulties in his relationships. Social workers have to be ready to help on both levels. Some clients are easy to help, some very difficult, some may be relatively self-supporting, while others, less mature, are extremely dependent and demanding. Some may only need temporary assistance, while others have been so badly damaged by life that they will always need some measure of support though, given that, they may be able to manage quite well. Some may need other kinds of help, for example, psychiatric treatment or residential care or a cure for loneliness, and the social worker will refer them to the appropriate agency if possible, but if the right kind of help is not available she will do the best she can without it. Some help is better than none at all.

Success in social work does not necessarily mean a complete cure, nor will social workers always succeed in solving or even lessening the problems brought to them. Indeed it may be part of their task to help certain clients to accept the fact that some problems are insoluble and that human suffering cannot be eradicated. But even when there is little that they can do to alter some situations, concern for the client may itself bring him comfort. Often they will be able to relieve stress at some point and this may be just enough to enable the client to cope with the rest of his problem. This is illustrated by the detailed case records in the following chapters.

C

CHAPTER III

SOCIAL WORKERS IN ACTION: MRS WHITE AND GORDON

THIS is a record by a hospital medical social worker (almoner). It shows how the situation developed at different dates over a period of two months and then summarizes subsequent developments. It is a record of work with a teenager threatened with blindness. He and his widowed mother both required help in adjusting to the boy's disability and its consequences. It illustrates how the almoner adapted her way of working to meet their different needs; this meant to stand by Gordon in his efforts to come to terms with his blindness and to support his mother who was bewildered by the enormity of the affliction and felt helpless through not knowing how to behave towards her son.

December 29th. The consultant physician asked me to see Gordon White, aged sixteen, who has an incurable eye disease. He can distinguish light and dark but for practical purposes he is blind. Last night Dr Fisher explained to Gordon that he would not improve and had told him that the almoner would discuss change of work with him. Dr Fisher will talk to Mrs White as soon as she visits next. Gordon may go home in a few days' time and come to see the eye consultant as an out-patient to be examined for entry on the blind register.

The ward sister told me that Gordon had had a restless night, waking frequently in tears and needing a great deal of comfort from the night staff. This morning, however, he was very off-hand, cracking jokes, almost as though nothing had happened. The sister thought he must be under considerable strain and the sooner he could talk about his future the better. She would send Mrs White to me as soon as Dr Fisher had seen her.

Gordon is an exceptionally tall, handsome boy, who greeted me soberly as soon as I introduced myself. He was expecting me. His first comment was that he wished his mother did not have to know about this. He did not think she would be able to take it. His eyes filled with tears which he hastily stifled and seemed to welcome my more general questions about his family and work. He explained that he is an only child whose father died when he was an infant. He has many very old relatives living nearby, his mother being the youngest of a large family. Since leaving school a year ago he has worked for a firm of draughtsmen. He obviously cannot go on working there, but shrugged help-lessly saying he had no idea what else to try. I agreed that this was a question needing a great deal of thought and not one about which any quick decisions could be made.

With no prompting from me, Gordon went on to speak with angry protest about missing his football, table tennis and athletics. He described how he has been losing at table tennis—a vivid description of being teased at missing the ball and not knowing whether to mention his eye trouble or not. He could imagine it sounding pretty feeble, as if he were making excuses. I agreed it was an awkward dilemma. He made his point about missing sport very emphatically.

Gordon then came back to whether his mother need know and finally commented that he supposed she guessed any-way. He seemed relieved that I intended to see her as soon as she had talked to Dr Fisher. We agreed that I would need to see him some more after he had gone home. There was too much to think about to decide anything quickly and it was too hard to think about blindness for any length at a stretch. I enquired about how he would get to hospital to see me. He angrily insisted that I need not worry about that. I supposed people would offer to help him and it would make

him feel cross. He agreed gloomily. We left it that I would
see his mother and fix a time for him to come to see me.

December 30th. Mrs White came to the office. She is a
dowdily dressed woman in late middle age, talking in a flat
expressionless way. She spoke haltingly, frequently shrug-
ging, and her sentences trailing off. She had talked to Dr
Fisher last night and although she had visited Gordon afterwards they had spoken of his home-coming, not about
his blindness. Mrs White spoke of the terrible thing this was
for Gordon, how it had ruined his life and how she wondered
why something like this had happened to Gordon who had
everything to live for. She suspected this might happen, because their general practitioner had tried to warn her, but she
was unable to believe it was true.

Mrs White said she was widowed when Gordon was four
and had worked to support him with the help of her relatives
who live nearby. She has been worried about work for herself recently as she found she could not keep up with the
factory work she had been doing since her husband's death.
She was lucky to find an alternative job in an office with
kind employers so that she will have an income for her
later years. This job is in a neighbouring town with fares
to pay but light and easy.

I told Mrs White of the services that were available for
Gordon as a blind person. She knew something of this already but protested that she would not want to think of him
with blind people and certainly would not let him go away
anywhere for training. She pointed out in a simple un-
ashamed fashion that he was 'her world' and she had nothing to live for except him.

Mrs White enquired about Gordon's financial position. He
still has pay from his work and sickness benefit but she will
have to tell his boss that he cannot return and she doubts if
she can support him on her wage of £7 a week. I told her
that the National Assistance Board could be approached
once his pay stops. She will tell me what happens about this.

Mrs White said she was relieved that I would explain

things to Gordon. We arranged that Gordon would come to see me on the same day as he comes to see the eye consultant, Dr Page. She would like to see me again after she has taken Gordon home. She gave the impression of feeling cut off from him, perhaps even frightened of being alone with him, though she did not openly admit this.

January 4th. Mrs White came by appointment. She complained of feeling depressed and of a barrier between her and Gordon. She would like to know what terms the doctor used when he told him he would not recover but she cannot bring herself to ask Gordon. He seems happy a great deal of the time and she does not want to be responsible for reminding him about his problem by introducing the matter in conversation.

Gordon is staying with Mrs White's sister at present as otherwise he would be alone all day while she is at work. When he first left hospital he slept in their flat and went to his aunt's day by day. Since the weather has been so bad they decided he had better stay at his aunt's place. Although she did not say so, I think she is relieved not to be alone with Gordon because she does not know what to say to him.

Mrs White had a great deal to say about the enormous tragedy of all this, speaking with some anger about a fellow employee who is upset because his seventy-year-old mother has gone blind. While she thinks this is a bad problem for them to have, she resents being told about something that falls so far short of Gordon's troubles.

We discussed whether Mrs White was willing for me to go ahead with plans for a worker in the local authority welfare department to see her and Gordon. She wished they could just stay as they are without having to think about the future, but acknowledged that for everyone's sake active steps must be taken. She would be glad if I would go ahead with this.

I told Mrs White that I wanted to see her, not only to ask about registration with the local authority but also because she seemed to be so distressed about Gordon. She said that she appreciated this very much as there was no place she could talk about it. Although she seemed to be both angry and miserable she was not forthcoming about her feelings and was, I felt, forbidding me to get too close. Nevertheless she co-operated in making a further appointment. Gordon is to see Dr Page and me on January 9th and Mrs White would like to see me after that.

We had a discussion about whether she would like to come to the clinic with Gordon or not. On the one hand she is nervous about his going out alone, but at the same time she hesitates to speak to the doctor in his presence. If she did not come with him she would like to think he had a car. He would be impatient of this but she would like to insist that he have it. I thought it useful to encourage any positive steps she felt she could take as Gordon's mother and agreed to order a car if she decided not to come with him herself. She wanted to think about this and telephone to me.

January 8th. Mrs White telephoned. She has decided it would not be justified to take time off from work to accompany Gordon tomorrow, so I arranged for a car to bring him.

January 9th. Gordon was seen in the eye clinic by Dr Page who thought there was some slight sign of improvement in his vision. He did not, at this point, want to make a final decision about his registration as a blind person giving his opinion that although cure was impossible some improvement might be hoped for. He therefore thought no decisive moves ought to be made at present, while he observes Gordon at monthly intervals. Gordon complained to him of feeling bored so the doctor wondered if I could help him do something about this. He would like him to be happily occupied but not doing anything too physically strenuous. If he is very careful crossing roads, Gordon should be able to travel by bus. Gordon asked him about this.

I saw Gordon today and again the following week. I wrote to Mrs White explaining that Dr Page wanted Gordon to wait a while before going ahead with work plans and confirming that the doctor had said that Gordon could travel by bus. Offered Mrs White an appointment for January 18th.

During our two interviews Gordon made good use of opportunities to discuss his situation. He mostly sat slouched in his chair, irritable and discontented and protesting quite belligerently at times. I tried to take up whatever he was saying to encourage him to go on and speak his mind. He had a lot to say about one doctor saying one thing and another something different. I agreed that this was what had happened and it was confusing and irritating. He wished he knew where he stood and had heard his mother saying the same thing to his aunts. I sympathized about having to wait for something so very important.

Another discontent was what to do with himself. He repeated at greater length his experience of being teased for losing at table tennis. People he used to be able to beat comfortably can now give him ten points and still win. He mimicked himself saying in a joking, deprecating way that he couldn't see the ball and the others mocking him—'Listen to White, full of excuses.' I had the impression that all this was fairly good-humoured but Gordon could not take this well-intentioned banter. He has only been back to his club once since leaving hospital. He does not want to go just to talk. If the others are playing that is all he thinks about too. He went on to tell me that he won the local junior championship last year. The club was beaten by a team from a neighbouring town in the finals but this year he was sure they would have won if he had been in the team. As it is he thinks they will be beaten again. He went on to tell me about his football activities, his training and his half hope that he could be a professional. He knew this was never certain but it was the job he would have liked best to do. He was close to tears about this and accepted my sympathy in quite a simple fashion. We discussed listening to sports reports on the radio and having people to read to him from the newspapers. He likes being read to but hates asking his family to do it, though they seem to do it willingly enough.

Gordon complained of feeling ill at ease with his mother and aunts who fuss about him and help him unnecessarily.

We had a long discussion about this. He recognized that being an only child among a lot of women he has to put up with fussing in any event. He paid less attention to it when he could see but now they make him feel like a baby. We recognized how uncomfortable this is and the fact that mothers and aunts tend to act this way. He dislikes too the way his mother and aunts tell everybody about him. He hates pity and special consideration. We agreed that he is receiving a lot of this and is having his temper sorely tried.

Gordon also told me that his mother gets on his nerves by giving him too many things. This is a problem not specially connected with his blindness but it is being brought home rather forcefully at present. Every Easter it has been his custom to have a new suit. His mother proposes to go ahead and get him one this Easter as usual. He discussed his dilemma about this. On the one hand he likes clothes and likes to look fashionable, but he feels guilty about his mother having to make special efforts for him as she is a widow and not earning much.

We discussed ideas about what he could do with himself while he waits about for the next few months. He discarded the idea of swimming with an instructor as it is too cold and he only likes the beach, not the baths. He showed more interest in having someone outside the family read to him about sport but was apprehensive about having some elderly person who would fuss over him and expect him to be interested in things he did not understand. He preferred that I did not do anything special about any of this for the time being.

As he was leaving at the end of the second interview Gordon, who knew that I was seeing his mother the following day, asked me not to tell her that he was feeling fed up with her. I told him I would talk to her about arranging his financial affairs as she would have to know about this as he is only 16. He accepted this. I told him I was very careful in a situation like this not to discuss his private affairs with his mother nor her private affairs with him. Rather awkwardly he said he thought this was a very good idea and useful that it could work like this.

January 18th. Mrs White came. I gave her opportunities to say she was confused about the medical position. She responded in a rather depressed fashion knowing that conflicting opinions had been given but not reacting very strongly about it. She said that Gordon told her his sight was better and that he could go about on his own without needing the hospital car. She did not altogether believe this until she had my letter. She thinks that Gordon sometimes jokes and says silly things about his blindness, so she does not know what the exact position is. I had the impression that she was willing to let things drift for the time being, perhaps even relieved that no big decisions had to be made.

I enquired about Mrs White's financial position. Gordon's firm has stopped paying him now and has returned his cards to Mrs White. She would like to try and get an extra allowance for him. His clothes are very expensive and he eats far more than most normal adults. His sickness benefit (32s 6d) goes on his pocket money, dry cleaning and shoe repairs. Gordon offers her his cheque every week but she finds that she needs to give back that amount of money to him in any event so does not take it in the first place. I offered to enquire what hope there was of extra N.A.B. allowance. She would like to know exactly what to do before she asks for further time off to attend to this.

When I asked again about Mrs White's own financial position she quickly and defensively said that she had told me once before that she earned £7 a week. I enquired if she also had a widow's allowance at which she made a long speech about never having had any help from anywhere, never having broken the law, nor taken anything she was not entitled to. I commented that she did not have to discuss her affairs with me, but I thought she was unhappy and in difficulties and I would like to help if I could. Mrs White then explained that Gordon is illegitimate. It was difficult for her to speak about this and it was clear that she has years of pent-up resentment about it, which is largely unexpressed. She pointed out several times that she has made no pretence with the taxation authorities about her true position, has had no allowance or concessions to distinguish her from a single woman, though she calls herself Mrs White. Gordon knows nothing of this, though she expects that he may have to some time. She has had offers of marriage provided Gordon were cared for elsewere, but she decided that Gordon was her first responsibility and had to stay with her.

At no time did Mrs White speak easily of this matter. She was defensive, returning briefly to the subject and dropping it again. She was obviously uncertain of my attitude and not sure that she should have told me.

January 23rd. Mrs White came to discuss the information I had from the National Assistance Board. Because Gordon is sixteen and has been at work he is considered an independent adult and his mother's circumstances are irrelevant. Their allowance for a sixteen-year-old is 32s and Gordon is therefore already 6d over. Special rates for blind people only apply after registration. He would probably get help with fares to hospital, prescription charges and any major expense, but no addition to his regular living allowance. When he is 18 he would be allowed part of the household rent.

Mrs White was quietly bitter about this information. She went on to comment with increasing spirit that she has never got help from anywhere with Gordon so should not be surprised that she could not have any now. I suggested that we should go thoroughly into her own financial position to see if she had a case for approaching a voluntary fund which would not have the kind of rules that the N.A.B. has. She co-operated enthusiastically in this.

Income

	£	s	d
Mrs White's wages (after deductions)	7	9	0
Gordon's sickness benefit	1	12	6
	9	1	6

Expenditure

	£	s	d
Rent	1	1	0
Gas, electricity, coke		17	0
Mrs White's fares		12	6
Insurance		3	6
Allowance to Mrs White's sister for Gordon's food	1	5	0
Mrs White's lunches		15	0
Milk		4	8
Groceries	1	5	0
Meat	1	5	0
Fruit and vegetables		10	0
	7	18	8

This budget does not take into account laundry, cleaning, repairs, pocket money for Gordon or saving for clothes. £1 5s. 0d. paid to relatives is to cover Gordon's lunch, tea and sometimes supper, while Mrs White is at work. She does not think this covers the cost but cannot afford more. The household where he spends the day consists of two sisters and a brother, all single, and all pensioners. She would like to be able to provide more milk for Gordon and has in fact been managing on this budget by going without her lunches. She provides Gordon's food herself at the week-ends.

We agreed that an approach to N.A.B. should be made for what little help might be got. Gordon has to apply himself so she will discuss this with him. She thought they had no case as yet for asking for special help with clothing, though this will become necessary as the year goes on.

We also agreed that I would approach the Samaritan Fund on her behalf and telephone her at work when we knew the result. We had some discussion about Mrs White's feelings at having told me about herself. She hoped I did not imagine that she concealed the facts in any illegal way. She kept insisting that it was old history now and that she had adap-

ted herself to it. I had the impression that she was torn
between wanting and not wanting to talk about it. In discussing future appointments I offered to see her on a
Saturday morning so that she need not take time off from
work. Her response to this was that she would never
use anybody's Saturday time for work. Her present job
is a five-day one, the first she has ever had, so she realizes
how valuable it is to people not to have to work on Satur-
days. I thought she was at least partly not wanting to see
me, and partly wanting to see how much trouble I would
go to for her.

January 24th. Mrs White telephoned to say that her boss
had enquired progress after her visit to me yesterday and was
extremely angry to hear that an additional living allowance
was not forthcoming from the National Assistance Board. He
planned to have the matter taken up by his M.P. Mrs White
thought she ought to let me know about this in case it influenced what I was doing. I encouraged her to go on talking about this as it was very plain that the words she was
quoting as her boss's were really her own. I acknowledged
that she was very angry at not being helped in the way she
expected. She emphasized that she was not angry with me
but just angry in general. I thanked her for letting me know
all this but said that I would go ahead with approaching
the Samaritan Fund whatever her boss was doing about the
N.A.B.
About an hour later Mr Moore, Mrs White's employer,
phoned. He gave the impression of making great efforts to
sound calm and reasonable. He thought it a bad situation
that a woman in Mrs White's position could get no help
with a problem like this. He wondered if there was anything
he could do. I told him I would be happy to discuss this
with him but first I would need Mrs White's specific permission to do so. He saw the sense of this and we arranged
to speak again when we had both spoken to Mrs White.

January 25th. I discussed Mrs White's financial position

with the secretary of the Samaritan Fund. He agreed to 10s. a week pocket money being offered to Gordon and 10s. a week allowance to be given to Mrs White until a definite decision is made about application for registration.

I telephoned Mrs White to tell her this. She received the news in a very curious way—a mixture of mock surprise and pleasure. Somewhat sarcastically she said she was expecting me to telephone at any time to tell her that no help was available. She went on to sound more pleased in a less complicated way giving the impression that the size of the grant was irrelevant. It was the fact of being given something which had made such an impression on her. She repeated 'Fancy them agreeing to help.'

Mrs White said that it was all right for me to talk to Mr Moore. He spoke to her about telephoning and she was surprised and gratified that the hospital had behaved so correctly. I could talk to him about her financial position quite freely but she would not like me to mention anything personal about her.

There had been an interruption to Gordon's appointments at the hospital because he was in bed with 'flu. Mrs White reported that he was now better and we made an appointment for him to come on January 29th.

I telephoned Mr Moore who no longer seemed angry about N.A.B. and pleased that the hospital was helping.

January 29th. Gordon came. He has not been out much because of his bad cold but spent some time telling me about the few outings he has had with friends. He has been to a club dance and to a youth club party for the younger children. Some of his friends were helping so he went along and talked to them. His family is reading all he wants to hear from the newspapers and he has been to the homes of some of his friends to play pop records. We discussed whether he wanted further activity but in the end he decided not. He will be out most evenings now he thinks and has plenty to interest him. He went on almost in tears to tell me about a friend getting a new scooter. If he was still at work he would have

a scooter too but there is no question of it now. He shrugged
off any sympathy about this.

I told Gordon of my arrangement with his mother that
we would pay him 10s. per week pocket money and asked if
he would come to the hospital each week to collect it. He
seemed very pleased about this, commenting that he would
not mind coming up for this purpose combining it with a
visit to me. In quite a challenging way he said that he hates
coming to the hospital and would not come at all if his
mother did not make him. Coming to see me, however, was
a bit easier than going to the doctor. We agreed that
nobody came to hospital for pleasure. It was usually for
something you wished you didn't have to think about.

We discussed his application to the N.A.B. for fares and
prescription charges. He asked what he would have to do
and what would happen. He clearly did not like the idea of
this and said he would like to discuss it with his mother
before deciding. She had mentioned it to him but he was not
too sure about it. We agreed that if he got N.A.B. money for
fares and prescriptions this would not mean extra cash in his
pocket but would save his mother having to give him money
for these purposes.

February 1st. Mrs White came to arrange for the payment
of her allowance. She made quite a speech about being so
unexpectedly helped. She felt that something new had come
into her life. She said that she hoped that she could still
come to see me because I was the only person who knew fully
about Gordon and she had to admit she found him pretty
difficult. This was the first time that Mrs White had frankly
complained about Gordon's behaviour. She did not show
much anger but joked about him. She made a funny story
describing the way she read the football results to him. She
gets all the names wrong, and because she does not understand what she is reading says things in a meaningless way
apparently that annoys Gordon. She mimicked the angry,
disparaging things he says to her. We laughed about this but
I commented that it was no doubt amusing for the spectator

to see this sort of thing but it must be pretty trying to put up with day in, day out. We discussed Gordon's age and the way boys of 16 tend to be critical of parents.

Mrs White spoke at length about the tragedy of blindness for Gordon and all the things it will spoil for him. She complained how difficult it was to bear the uncertainty while they waited for the doctor's verdict. She does not notice any improvement herself and neither does his aunt. He is very clumsy, making an awful mess over meals and so on. She described her distress as she watched this and does not think that anyone can appreciate what it all means to her. She wondered if she would come to the doctor with him next week so she could ask the doctor herself what all this is about. She sounded less depressed and more aggressive than usual as she said this and I encouraged her to do it.

February 12th. Both Mrs White and Gordon came, after Gordon's appointment with Dr Fisher. When I went to the waiting-room Mrs White made to send Gordon in first but I said I preferred to see her first in case she wanted to get back to work. She told me that Gordon objected to her coming with him today but she had insisted. It was not so much that she wanted to see Dr Fisher as fearing the traffic for him. To her mind his eyesight is no better than it was. At the clinic she did not automatically go in with Gordon until Dr Fisher invited her to follow. He did not say anything except that Gordon should continue seeing Dr Page and coming to see me. She spoke of Gordon's continuing irritability with her, sighing and adding that she realized that he was bound to be like this. He was particularly trying while laid up with his 'flu but is better now that he is able to get out more. I asked if she had discussed with Gordon his application to the N.A.B. She said that they had talked about it and she wanted him to apply.

When Gordon came in he told me first of a recent outing with a friend to a football match. They drove up to Twickenham and stayed in London overnight. He couldn't see in any detail but he enjoyed being with his friends. He spoke of other things he and his friends used to do together last summer. I enquired how Gordon's friends took his disability. He spoke with a great exasperation of other people's reactions. He mimicked the local women in gossiping huddles about him and the way people want him to talk about his eyes. The boys he knows well do not pursue the matter when they get an abrupt answer from him. I commented that I supposed they wanted to know about him if he was going about with them. He supposed this was so but wished nothing had to be said on the subject. He blames his mother and aunts for the local interest in him, particularly his aunts as his mother is at work all day with little opportunity for gossiping.

Gordon went on to tell me in some detail about how a man he knew was killed in a scooter accident last week. We agreed how shocking it is to know somebody who is suddenly killed. He told me in great detail how it all happened and then described a narrow squeak of his own. We agreed that the traffic problem was really serious and we could see why mothers were worried about young people being out.

We discussed how Gordon was managing everyday things. He made a long attempt to describe to me what it was like not seeing things clearly. He ended in some exasperation by saying it was too difficult to make someone else picture what it was like. I agreed I found it hard to imagine myself. It seems, however, that he is in no danger of bumping into anything big though very fast moving traffic is a danger and he is very careful about it. I was impressed that Gordon really did take this problem seriously but I could see that his mother probably does not think so because he will not listen to her comments on the matter and brushes it aside as fussing. He is learning to distinguish people by general outline, walk and voice. In his opinion he is not seeing any worse but is not seeing any better either.

I asked Gordon about the National Assistance Board and whether he was satisfied with his mother's view about it. He said there had been some talk but asked if I thought she agreed. I said I thought she did, so he said he might as well get on with it. I helped him fill up the form and sent it in for him with an accompanying letter.

February 19th. The National Assistance officer rang up. He has seen Gordon and is so impressed with his size and food requirements that he has asked permission from the area officer to make an 'exceptional circumstances grant'. This will be 1s per day, that is 7s per week, less 6d as his sickness benefit is 6d over their basic allowance anyway. Gordon will have a book for 6s 6d per week extra allowance and will have all fares and prescription charges refunded.

Summary to March 8th

Gordon

Gordon has been seen again by Dr Page who told me that the very slight improvement in his eyesight seems to have halted and after his next visit he will probably take steps towards registering him as blind.

Gordon has come to see me weekly. The main problem looked at was his new poverty. He is very keen on style and fashion and disgruntled that he has to wear last year's clothes which are shabby and too tight. He would like a new suit and the latest style in shoes. He cannot get these for himself, does not want to ask his mother because he knows she cannot manage it and with angry scorn said that he knew the N.A.B. man would not even listen. I agreed that N.A.B. would not help him with the particular things he wanted but we finally agreed that they might well help him with some jeans for everyday wear so that he can save his best suit. After two discussions he settled for this and the application went off very smoothly.

Gordon and I had planned that he would call at the office each week on his way to my office to collect his 10s. After he had done this once he asked me if he could sign for his money in my room instead of in the general office as he felt silly having to be helped in front of other people who were

D

waiting. He thought it was all right for me to help him because I knew what it was all about. I agreed to this and we followed that procedure from then on.

Gordon complained quite often about how his mother fusses him. Even before his eyes were bad she used to sit up for him to come in in the evenings and always wanted to know where he had been. I enquired about how other people's mothers acted. He agreed with a sigh that they are all the same. He seemed to get somewhat more indulgent about this.

Gordon continued to speak about his impatience with people's curiosity and concern for him. I noticed that while he told me very frequently that he did not like speaking about his eyes he often volunteered comment to me about how much he could and could not see and his belief that there was some slight improvement. I think I may be the only person to whom he can speak about his eyes.

In our last interview we forecast that the problem of work was approaching and that getting started will be hard. Gordon has lost much of his restlessness and partly enjoys his idle existence—he stays in bed until late in the mornings, goes to his aunt's in the afternoon and out with his friends most evenings.

Mrs White

Mrs White has mainly discussed her inability to talk with Gordon about his eyes. She wants to know about them but Gordon is so rude to her when she tries that she gives up. She accompanied him to his last appointment to Dr Page, half hoping for a word with the doctor but as she was not specifically invited in she lacked the courage to take the initiative to ask. Again I acknowledge the naturalness of her wish for information, and supported her belief in her right to it. I said that even if Gordon were prepared to talk to her about it I thought it was quite proper for her to want to know direct from the doctor himself. On the next occasion when I was seeing Gordon after the clinic Mrs White telephoned to say that when Gordon had gone into my room she had gone back to the clinic and asked to see the doctor. They had had a talk about Gordon and she now felt she knew what was happening.

In our last interview during this period Mrs White seemed to feel much better at the way she and Gordon were managing. She feels that the worst is past and that they can talk to each other better. She is not so put off by his irritability and even reprimands him if she thinks he has gone too far and is too rude to her. We forecast that when the time comes to take action about registering him they will have to think about his future and will probably feel unsettled and upset again. Just at present, however, they are getting along quite comfortably.

Here we can see the way in which the social worker in hospital can offer help in facing chronic disability. She is part of the medical team and as such has some responsibility for helping the patient to persevere with treatment. She plays her part in sharing with the ward sister the impact of the doctor's verdict on Gordon's eyes and of helping Mrs White to go back and question the doctors when she was diffident about approaching them. She is also the link for Gordon between medical care and life in the community and in his family. She is called in here to meet Gordon's need for help in becoming accustomed to his blindness and in matching the medical diagnosis to suitable plans for work and leisure. Because Mrs White and Gordon are so important to each other Mrs White, too, is affected by his loss of eyesight and needs help in adjusting to the changed situation at home.

Blindness normally excites compassion more than any other physical disability. When the blind person is a teenager full of zest for life, strong feelings are aroused which make people act in an exaggerated way. Everybody wants to help Gordon, to do things for him and to make him happy. We see this with Gordon's family and friends: his mother is so upset that she cannot see how to behave towards him; his aunts in their anxiety overwhelm him with well-meaning attempts to do things for him and they relieve their feelings by chattering to the neighbours; his friends are shy in approaching him, so for Gordon the stress of other people's reactions to him is added to the problem of becoming blind.

Because Gordon was enabled to talk freely in this way, we have no need to speculate about where his need for help lay. He told the social worker what it was that troubled him most: it was his rage and frustration at having to be helped —the thing that hit him harder than the inability to play games or keep his job. It was the normal reaction for anyone of his age. At the time when he was feeling his way towards adult independence and towards a suitable masculine relationship with his mother and his aunts he was forced back on their help in a way that made him feel 'babied'. The normal adolescent problems of a fatherless boy were increased in an overwhelming way. For this sixteen-year-old there could be no solution; he could only be helped to bear it and to reshape his life within the limitations of little or no sight.

The main thing that Gordon needed at this moment was someone who could stand outside his emotional upheaval and let him talk about what was happening to him; someone who would allow him to mourn for his lost eyesight and give him time to come to terms with all that the loss implied; someone who would try to understand how much he hated being helped and being the object of attention and pity. Recognizing this, the social worker set out to show him that she would try to understand with him what blindness meant to him. By her acceptance of his misery she demonstrated that she would try to help him without the personal involvement or the embarrassing sympathy that he dreaded: she could stand outside the emotional upheaval and help him to talk about what was happening to him. As a result, he could let loose some of the tumultuous feelings that were churning around inside him. Her acknowledgement that this was not something about which a quick decision could be made and her offer to take all the time he needed to talk it over enabled him to begin to think more calmly. He was assured by her attitude rather than by words that no plans for his future would be made over his head, but that she would support him and his mother in planning something that he wanted to do to earn his living, as long as it was medically advisable. This was sealed at the end of the first interview by their joint agreement that blindness was 'too hard to think about for too long at a time'. In telling him that she realized that 'people will offer to help him and that this will madden him' the social worker confirmed that she understood his repugnance at being conspicuous and at having to be helped publicly and that she knew the sort of things that he would have to face. In these ways she identified herself as willing to try to understand his troubles and his feelings about them and had begun to develop a relationship within which he could feel free to discuss his disability and to find a way of living with it.

The social worker demonstrated in her handling of the offer of pocket money her recognition of Gordon's wish to be independent. To be given money by itself could have merely reinforced Gordon's fury at having to be given to, but by the arrangement that he could call to collect it and stay on to talk with her he was enabled to make use of casework help. In this skilful combination she acknowledged his real need for money, both in itself and as a token of independence.

Later Gordon could describe in more detail how irritated he was by the way his aunts gossiped about him. He could tell of his discomfort at his friends' timid efforts to approach him and of his dislike of pity, and he received the social worker's assurance that it was reasonable to feel like this. The result was that Gordon reported later that he was getting about more and enjoying people's company. He had used the social worker as somebody whom he could trust to listen without being either over-sentimental or critical while he sorted out his ideas. He did not want advice. He behaved more freely once he had found an outlet for his uncomfortable feelings.

By the end of the period there were substantial changes.

Gordon had been helped to continue treatment. He had been able to feel independent by having some money of his own and to accept some measure of dependence, for example, in allowing his mother's stumbling efforts to read the football results. He had also resumed contacts with some of his friends and could enjoy football and 'pop' music in their company. Above all, he had begun to slow down the pace of life to something within his compass. He had begun to learn to tolerate himself and be more patient in his relationship with others.

For Mrs White the immediate problem was her acute distress for Gordon. She wanted to protect and help him but was afraid of doing the wrong thing. She was not sure even how to speak to him. Their old relationship was well-established but now she needed help in finding a new way of thinking about Gordon and talking to him. She had also the practical problem of making ends meet.

Mrs White was a fiercely independent person. She had struggled for years to maintain standards and to clothe and feed this young giant. She was resentful that no financial help had been given and thus too angry to ask for it. In the complexity of her feelings she was depressed and inarticulate. She needed the assurance that she was still of use to Gordon who was 'her world'. The social worker's job, therefore, was to concentrate on Mrs White's relationship with Gordon, her sense of responsibility towards him and her longing to be the person who could support him through this tremendous difficulty. The social worker had to break through Mrs White's reluctance to accept casework help and her depression about her problems before she could be of use. She began to establish a relationship by telling Mrs White that she realized that Gordon's loss of eyesight created a painful situation for her, too. She showed Mrs White that she recognized her as a person needing help in her own right, not just as part of the hospital's treatment of Gordon. She reinforced this by drawing her into consultations with the doctors, from which she had felt excluded, and by emphasizing her role as Gordon's mother in the whole treatment process and plans for the future. This insistence on Mrs White's own needs and her importance as a person reassured her so strongly that she could confide the nagging guilt that she had not been able to speak about up to now; when the social worker's response was to propose a plan to ease Mrs White's economic difficulties she was glad to accept it. Mrs White's security in this relationship was finally sealed by the social worker's refusal to discuss her affairs without permission and by her careful checking with Mrs White of the information she would wish to be kept confidential. The dual acknowledgment of the tangible and intangible problems which Mrs White faced—her real need of money and her resentment about asking for it, her longing to be understood and her fear of allowing anyone to know of her failure reinforced her energies and freed her to begin to work out ways of dealing with them herself. Mrs White had been helped to talk about her pain and anger in relation to Gordon. The feelings which had overwhelmed her and prevented her from acting in her usual way, had been modified. As the strain on her lessened by sharing her distress with the social worker, Mrs White began to see how she could resume her role as the mother of a fatherless adolescent boy. She still felt awkward and unhappy about his blindness but she could tolerate it more easily and was less tiresomely protective about him. She still became annoyed by his irritability but could now correct him without feeling guilty when he went too far. After releasing some of her anger about the past, she readily accepted the social worker's offer of financial help, both as a badly needed supplement to her earnings and as a token of the almoner's understanding of her need.

For both Mrs White and Gordon there was the added stress of the uncertainty about the prognosis. The social worker relieved this, as far as it could be relieved, by acknowledging the extra strain it was for them and by practical measures of help. She used the opportunity to help Mrs White and Gordon to talk together about this. There were individual problems which they could not share at this stage, but part of the social worker's aim was to draw them together so that with her help they could begin to discuss the results of Gordon's blindness without embarrassment.

Her knowledge of this drive towards independence had to be demonstrated as well as told. This was achieved by showing that in their relationship with her the Whites could acknowledge their needs and yet retain their right to think and plan for themselves. She would smooth the way and support them but she would not intrude on their responsibility for finding their own solution.

In working towards this the social worker used her understanding of the strong need of every normal person to be independent, to come and go as he pleases and to make his own decisions. She also used her knowledge that physical handicap highlights all of these characteristics; that the fear of losing independence and the indignity of having to accept help with simple, everyday actions generate anger which is accentuated by helplessness to alter the situation. The usual reaction of people to handicap is to offer assistance, which is sometimes really needed, but is often bitterly resented, either as an unwelcome reminder of the disability or as a frustration of the person's attempts to help himself. The common attitude is to urge patience and courage and 'to keep a stiff upper lip'. This is only to deny that person the right to have feelings about his loss of function, to mourn his lost independence. The social worker must know how to offer help which will give a handicapped person the chance to come to terms with his disability. Newly disabled people need to be allowed to grieve for their lost freedom and they can normally only come to terms with disability through first being able to express anger and resentment. To deny them this would be to jeopardize their chances of reinstatement as self-respecting people in society. To learn to adapt to handicap is a daunting task which can rarely be appreciated by anyone who is not disabled. However much time is needed is legitimately spent in helping a disabled person to come to his own compromise solution. Casework helped Gordon to overcome his anger and isolation and to resume some of his old interests. It was the first step in restoring his drive towards independence and to seeing himself as someone for whom life still held opportunities.

CHAPTER IV

SOCIAL WORKERS IN ACTION:
MR AND MRS UPTON

THIS is a record by a social worker in a family casework agency of his work over a period of a year with a family which had antagonized a number of workers and was itself becoming more and more entangled in its problems.

Mr Upton had never been a fit man but he had managed to keep in work as an unskilled house-painter until 1958 when he was thirty-nine. Then an old rheumatic heart condition flared up and made heavy physical exertion impossible. From that time he had had no regular work and his finances had got into a chaotic state. By May 1961 the family was in a crisis. Mrs Upton, who was thirty-four was pregnant and anaemic; the two older children, Thomas, aged eight and Mary, aged two, were always ailing; Alan was one year old and Josephine only two months. Debts had reached alarming proportions and grants from charitable funds had been absorbed with no noticeable improvement in the situation.

The disablement resettlement officer (D.R.O.), who had been trying to help Mr Upton to get back to work, decided that there were many issues involved and that Mr Upton was too much preoccupied with his family's affairs to think about work. Knowing that there were young children, he contacted the health visitor who agreed that both Mr and Mrs Upton were too anxious and unwell to begin to sort things out alone. She discussed the family's troubles with them on these lines and offered to contact an agency which would be able to spend time with them in sorting out what they could do. The Uptons accepted the offer and agreed that the health visitor should tell this agency about their present worries.

There were many complicating factors which the health visitor listed in a letter to the family casework agency. While it was true that Mr Upton had a defective heart, he was fit for work. After treating him for two years the doctor had asked the disablement resettlement officer to discuss plans for re-training. A course in making leather goods had been arranged but after only two months Mr Upton had been unfit to continue and was re-attending hospital. He seemed to prefer doing odd painting jobs to persevering with a training course that involved a daily journey. The health visitor wondered if the fact that his statutory allowance totalled as much as a basic wage removed the incentive to work. Another complication was Mr Upton's unrealistic attitute towards his debts; he insisted on keeping a motor cycle and sidecar, an electric drier and a television set—all on hire purchase—when his income was sufficient only to cover essentials. An Ascot water heater, for which he had completed payments, seemed a luxury but he would not part with it. Mrs Upton was thought 'not to be over-intelligent'; she was overshadowed by her husband who enjoyed a domestic role, but she managed well with the supervision of the health visitor and a daily home help when he was in hospital. Mr Upton was said to be a very worried man, feeling that his affairs were on top of him and that they could not afford another child. The family caseworker followed up the health visitor's verbal introduction by writing a letter to the Uptons saying that the health visitor had told him of the difficulties they were having, of his willingness to try to help them to sort these out and offering to call at a stated time or to see them at the office if they preferred. The letter added that if the social worker had no reply he would assume it was convenient to call. He had not received a reply and accordingly called at the suggested time.

The Uptons lived on the first floor of a block of local authority flats. It was a sparsely furnished home but well

kept and with signs that the family minded about their sur-
roundings being attractive. It was also clear that for some
time there had been little money available to provide re-
placements.

When the worker knocked it was Mr Upton who opened
the door. Mrs Upton hovered in the background, seeming
quite impassive except when her husband was out of the
room, when she managed to say a few words. Mr Upton
looked pale and unhealthy and was sulky, apathetic and
complaining. He saw money as the only solution to his problems: if only the D.R.O. or the National Assistance Board
had helped more it would have been different. He appreciated what a church fund had done and the free welfare foods,
but he still had debts. The worker agreed that his debts
must be worrying him a great deal and that he could see that
being so short of money was a big anxiety for him but he
thought there were other things on Mr Upton's mind—he
would be glad to hear more about his difficulties so as to
understand the whole position better. Mr Upton acknowledged that he would be glad of a chance to talk. He began at
once to do so at length; by the end of the interview he had
voiced a great deal of resentment about the various people
whom he had asked for help and whom he saw as having
made him feel 'only a cadger' for having asked. He seemed
to get some satisfaction from being listened to. Mrs Upton
just sat quietly most of the time, allowing her husband to do
the talking, but following intently all that was said. The
worker thought that little had been achieved at this interview
other than giving Mr Upton an opportunity to 'let off steam',
but arranged that he would call each week at a regular time
so that they could get to know each other better and begin
to plan ways of getting out of the difficulties.

At the second interview Mr Upton was less well, worrying
a great deal about his debts. The worker took the opportunity to learn the amount of these and the length of time
the hire purchase payments were due to continue. Mr Upton
was not quite clear exactly how much was owing, but it
seemed like something in the region of £50. As Mr Upton

discussed his debts, his intense need to keep his semi-luxuries became clear. Indeed it outweighed his anxiety at not being able to pay for them. The motor cycle was especially important to him: he had paid for the sidecar and for half of the cycle. He reasoned it out that he got exhausted travelling to work or training if he had to use public transport and it was his only means of taking the whole family out. He spoke of the motor bike with possessive passion. With less emotion Mr Upton explained that the electric drier was really no luxury because it heated the flat as well as drying the clothes and that the television was the only thing that kept the children quiet so that his wife could have a rest. It was clear that no logical discussion of ways and means was of any help to Mr Upton at this point.

During the same interview Mr Upton demonstrated how efficient he was at being 'Mum'. He feeds the baby, does the washing and takes the children to the clinic. He is also very good with his hands and proudly showed the cupboards, shelves and window-boxes he had made. He would like to take a training in watch-repairing so that he could work from home and, above all, he would like to live in the country. At this point Mrs Upton, who had said little, became animated and agreed that she had always longed for this, too.

Weekly interviews continued. In each interview the question of debts and especially the motor bike were the central theme. He was still paying frequent visits to other agencies who had given him financial help before and was becoming more and more frustrated at being refused. The worker never urged Mr Upton to part with his possessions and Mr Upton did not ask for money. The social worker discussed his worries in keeping the motor bike, hoping gradually to help him to formulate some plan that he could realistically carry out. Most of his ideas were unrealistic. He continued to be adamant that he must keep the motor bike and that he could not face going to do a course without it. The worker told Mr Upton that he knew he felt that it was the only way he could manage.

The next week Mr Upton had started a training course

but, after a month, he was taking time off because Mrs Upton and the children were ill. The social worker at the Industrial Rehabilitation Unit was doing all she could to keep his place open, but was facing the fact that he did not justify a vacancy when there was a waiting list. If he could not turn up regularly for training, it was unlikely that he could be regular in work, so that any training would be wasted. She discussed this with the caseworker who, in turn, took it up with Mr Upton. In this discussion the worker learned that the health visitor was in fact arranging for the two middle children to go to the day nursery to ease pressure on the household and to free Mrs Upton to do what her health allowed. Mr Upton was glad about this, but insisted that it did not solve his problem: he could not leave Mrs Upton and the baby. When pressed by the worker, he became acutely distressed and burst out that he could not face it, he was not strong enough.

By the next visit Mr Upton had been suspended. He was cheerful, busy with plans for taking the children to hospital for treatment. When her husband went out of the room, the worker asked Mrs Upton how she felt about Mr Upton's suspension. At last Mrs Upton asserted herself. She replied 'I'm that fed up; I wish I could run away from it all'. The worker agreed that it must be terribly worrying and discouraging for her. When Mr Upton returned the social worker discussed the fact that so many people were involved in different ways in trying to help the Uptons. He would like to be able to talk to them to see whether they were all working along the same lines and being as helpful as possible to the Uptons. The Uptons agreed.

A case conference was called at which the worker interpreted to his colleagues in other agencies the gist of what had been happening since he first met the family. Everyone recognized that Mr Upton made use of illness as a defence against leaving home to work and that he played off the agencies against each other in a fruitless effort to get someone 'on his side'. The agencies, by not working more closely together and having a common policy, had unwittingly connived at this and so had not been as helpful as they could have been. Mr Upton's need for attention was recognized as well as his real need for money. It was decided that to avoid confusion and to channel help more effectively any further financial help should be given through the family caseworker and that no further efforts would be made by other agencies to try to get him to work.

At the next visit the worker told the Uptons that all the agencies were anxious to be as helpful as they could; that they realized that it was unsatisfactory for Mr Upton to have to keep running round to so many places looking for help and had therefore decided that any further financial help would be given through him.

Following this Mr Upton asked directly for a grant of money to pay off outstanding instalments on the motor bike. The worker replied that he realized the problem of not having enough money was always on Mr Upton's mind, but that he knew from what he had told him that earlier grants had been made and had not solved the problem: he wanted to help him and felt that together they could get some better understanding of the way in which he really needed his help. Both Mr and Mrs Upton were furious and showed their feelings. Mr Upton declaring that if the worker couldn't give him money it was no use coming again: nobody cared for them—everybody was ready to tell them how they should manage, but they had no idea what it was like. Mrs Upton launched into an attack on the health visitor—she just came and talked and did nothing. The worker picked this up, saying that no doubt Mrs Upton felt that he, too, came and talked and did nothing to which Mrs Upton replied 'if the cap fits . . .'. The interview continued with Mrs Upton retiring into silence and Mr Upton maintaining his rigid attitude about his motor bike—he *had* to have it. The worker agreed that he knew this was his opinion and that Mr Upton was very angry with him because he seemed not to be helping. It was something important that they must talk more about when he came next week.

A week later Mr Upton was still in a militant mood and

Mrs Upton was sitting with her back turned when the worker
arrived, her attitude expressive. The worker began the interview by recalling how angry they had been at their last
meeting, adding that he thought it was right for them to tell
him so—he could only help them if they really told him what
they felt. At first Mr Upton denied being angry—it was just
that he'd been out of sorts. He needed a good deal of encouragement to express himself and to be assured that he
would not alienate the worker. Finally, he admitted that he
felt furious with everyone—the hospital, the National Assistance Board, the D.R.O. and the curate all made him feel
he ought to be at work; if they gave you money probably
they had the right to lecture you, but it made you feel you
weren't a real person. Even the visitor from one of the funds
had made them feel like that. She'd been good to them and
they'd wanted to please her; when they'd saved to buy shoes
for the child who was ill they'd been so proud, but she had
only said they shouldn't have spent the money that way because the child wouldn't be out of bed for some time yet.
They got no encouragement from anyone.

The worker agreed that Mr Upton must feel thoroughly
fed up with social workers who seemed not to understand
what he needed but just wanted to tell him what to do; he
thought Mr Upton must feel that he only came and talked
but things got no better. Mr Upton admitted that he had been
angry with him. The worker suggested he might be a bit cross
with himself too, for having to ask them all for help, adding
that he had been wondering how he really felt about not
being able to work. 'Worried and miserable' he replied, and
burst into tears. Mrs Upton was by this time standing in an
anxious way by her husband. The worker asked her what
she felt about it all. Mrs Upton said she got so worried about
him and not being able to help him that she couldn't think
of anything else—then she burst into tears too. She said
they must be awful people because everyone left them—her
sister and her aunt hadn't been near them for ages. Her aunt
had looked after her when she had her first baby. Now she
must have offended the aunt because it was so long since

she'd been to see them. No one seemed to be sending the children anything for Christmas; people just thought they were scroungers and not worth helping. The worker's reply was that he could understand that they felt awful about this constant asking for money and being refused—he could see it made them feel inferior and unwanted. The Uptons responded to this by agreeing that it was unbearable; they could not go on like this.

Mr Upton pulled himself together and described the different plans he had had to get his finances straight. He had even toyed with the idea of returning the bike, though clearly not very seriously. Mrs Upton chimed in that it was the last thing he'd got left for himself. As he began to review more objectively the sources of help, Mr Upton admitted that the National Assistance Board were reconsidering his allowance—they had told him that he might be entitled to additional benefits. He should have been to find out, but was so much afraid of another disappointment that he had kept away. The worker offered to find out for him, but Mr Upton decided he could now go himself. 'I feel I've got a lot off my chest since I went off at you—it makes all the difference to be able to tell you what I want to instead of wondering what you will expect me to say.' As the worker was leaving, Mr Upton rushed out of the room and returned with the doll's house which he was making as a Christmas present for the children. He showed it off with pride and was pleased with the worker's praise for his craftsmanship. The worker left after planning to return the next week to talk more about their plans.

After this the relationship between the Uptons and the social worker was much easier. The debts remained, but the Uptons began to work out more realistic ways in which to manage their affairs. Mr Upton still made sporadic efforts to seek concrete help and to react strongly against the people who refused it, but now he told the worker about these incidents. In discussion with him he could see something of his part in provoking people. There was the day when he called on the curate to ask for a few pounds. The curate had

E

reminded him of the money already given from church funds. Mr Upton had 'blown his top' and said no one should know better than he—he had to do the asking, the curate didn't think he enjoyed it, did he? The curate had told him he'd be better off doing an honest job to keep his family. Mr Upton was shaking with anger as he described the incident. The worker commented that it was plain that he hated going around cap in hand like this. Mr Upton agreed, saying 'but what else can I do—that's what makes me so angry. I used to think the curate was my best friend, but now he thinks I'm just scrounging.' This led to a discussion of other ways in which Mr Upton might help himself, ending in a plan for him to approach the hire purchase firms to ask them to accept a token sum each week until he got into work. Mr Upton became enthusiastic.

At the next visit he was thoughtful and commented to the social worker that it was strange how he never told him off, but made him feel he wanted to manage things better. The worker replied that he knew Mr Upton tried to make a go of it and that he lost his temper because it was hard to feel so helpless, but together they would find a way to get to grips with his problems. Mr Upton reported a satisfactory talk with the hire purchase firms. He wished he had been to them before, but he'd been sure they would not believe him. His self-respect was returning and with it his ability to assume responsibility for his family. He completed various repairs to the house, leaving Mrs Upton to manage the household affairs. As his morale improved his wife became happier and fitter.

A few weeks later Mr Upton asked if there was any hope of his getting training in carpentry: he reminded the worker that he had praised his work on the doll's house and shelves and said he would like to learn more about it. He enjoyed doing jobs about the house and would like to see if he could make a living at it. The worker promised to ask the D.R.O., while Mr Upton consulted his doctor about the suitability of this sort of work. The result was favourable and a vacancy on a training course in wood machining was obtained. Mr

Upton was excited. Telling the worker about his interview at the employment exchange, he said 'The D.R.O. was quite different from the last time I saw him; we had a joke together and he wished me luck. I feel I can do it now, but I'd like to feel you were around if I ran into difficulties again. The wife would like to see you, too'.

The worker agreed that although it all looked promising there might be pitfalls ahead and that he would call each week for a while just to hear how they were getting on.

For the Uptons the trouble is illness—a chronic, but not completely disabling condition that makes Mr Upton unfit for heavy work. It is aggravated by heavy weekly hire purchase commitments undertaken as reasonable while he was working, but now a nagging burden. Added to this is the attitude of society towards Mr Upton. As long as he was a man in poor health, managing to keep going, he was a respected citizen. The fact that his hire purchase arrangements were ambitious for a man with his earnings was his own business and no more questionable than those of his neighbours whose ideas flew higher than was prudent. He would even be considered far-sighted to buy a motor cycle and sidecar as the cheapest way of taking his family for outings. Whatever difficulties the Uptons might have were contained within the family.

When Mr Upton's illness prevents him from working and he is dependent on statutory allowances as his sole income the whole attitude is changed. He can no longer be allowed to indulge in hire purchase commitments which must be paid for from 'public money'. He is urged to get back to work as soon as he is pronounced fit and the social services are at his disposal to help him to do this. When he fails to make appropriate use of them he begins to become the object of criticism. He feels he has few comforts, but these he is urged to give up.

It is unfortunate for Mr Upton that his illness is unspectacular. A lost limb or blindness invite sympathy, but a man who appears to be whole and who is pronounced medically fit for light employment arouses only irritation when he does not do what seems to be a sensible thing. Mr Upton is sensitive about the invisible illness that makes him only half a worker and he is by no means sure of his adequacy as a provider for his family; the fact that the idea of light work implies something inferior to him becomes apparent only after he has failed to take advantage of the training offered. By then his ever-present debts are proof to him of his failure. He can see only one solution to his problems—to get someone to give him money. This provides a palliative but no permanent cure. Renewed requests have a twofold effect; society, already growing impatient, loses respect for Mr Upton; Mr Upton loses respect for himself. In his desperation and inadequacy he can see no way but to perpetuate this abortive pattern of 'begging'. The result is an ever-rising anger in the agencies against Mr Upton and in Mr Upton against the agencies. Added to the realistic problems of illness and debt is the stress set up between Mr Upton and society. Mr Upton is caught up in a vicious circle; his anger uses up all his energy and by himself he can see no way out.

Coming newly into it the social worker is in a position to see the pattern of the complex situation which Mr Upton has created and its effects on him and his family. The workers who were initially eager to help have become frustated by his failure to use their agencies appopriately, so that the social services, which should have been supporting him, have become a battle ground of Mr Upton's making. The social worker can see, too, that the ways in which Mr Upton has asked for help and the response which he has evoked have created humiliation for him; he has a real problem in lack of money, but underlying this is his desperate feeling of personal failure.

This coloured his views to the extent that he could not see the genuine goodwill shown by the officers of the social services. In approaching the employment exchange about a course which made him feel less than a man he saw the disablement resettlement officer as an ogre forcing him into an intolerable situation. Because Mr Upton was unable to express his fears, his reluctant response irritated the D.R.O. Once Mr Upton could begin to believe that he was a worthwhile person he could begin to behave like one. In looking forward to a training of his own choosing his whole outlook and demeanour was altered. Both he and the D.R.O. could approach the matter wholeheartedly and Mr Upton could see the D.R.O. as he really was—a jovial man, eager to see him succeed and competent to help.

In addition to getting some understanding of the situation, the social worker had to begin to consider what could be done about it; what strengths the Uptons had on which to build, and how Mr Upton could be helped to modify his angry attitutdes. Although both were people with difficulties in themselves, their marriage had survived under considerable strains; both had poor health, the children were frequently ailing and the pressure of mounting debts had increased steadily during the two years prior to their being referred to the family casework agency. They needed each other and were fond of their children, and, in spite of Mr Upton's erratic ways, they faced their difficulties together. The aim was to help Mr Upton to regain his self-respect and to resume his role as head of his family. His morale had been severely damaged by his experiences of seeking help and meeting refusal or rebuff. He had lost faith in the social services and, before he could begin to resume control of his affairs and to become a respected citizen, he needed to be shown that help could be offered in a way that was acceptable to him; that it was designed to build up his self-esteem through a realistic appraisal of his good and bad qualities and his potential skills as a breadwinner.

As a result of this appraisal, the social worker set out to build up a relationship with Mr Upton in which it would be apparent how he behaved when having to ask for help and how his behaviour antagonized the people he was asking to help him. Within this relationship Mr Upton could be accepted as the angry, inadequate man he felt himself to be, without the accompanying criticism which he expected.

Because he was accepted as a person worthy of consideration and the real nature of his dilemma was understood
Mr Upton could begin to look at himself and the effect he
was having on other people. With the worker's support he
could begin to modify his aggressive attitudes and to see his
balancing good qualities—his genuine affection and concern
for his wife and family, his skill as a handyman and his
determination to keep his home together in spite of the
odds against him. The vicious circle was broken and Mr
Upton was free to begin to recover his self-respect and to
work out a solution satisfying to himself and acceptable to
society.

The social worker's help consisted in his recognition of
Mr Upton's anger and helplessness in the complex situation
which he had created and his desperate need for restored
self-respect. Help was not offered in terms of money, although this was acknowledged as a real need, because
previous grants of money had been ineffective in solving
his problem, indeed had only increased his feelings of humiliation.

It was necessary for the social worker to demonstrate
respect for the Uptons by his whole attitude and actions, not
just in words. It was shown in his acknowledgement that
they had a problem and that they had conflicting feelings
about it; that they disliked 'being a problem' and having to
ask for help, and by refraining from the criticism which they
had grown to look on as inseparable from receiving help.
His respect for them was also shown in his concern lest they
should feel that the social workers they knew were talking
about them behind their backs. In discussing with them the
plans for a case conference he explained why he wanted to
consult his colleagues. It was a way of showing the Uptons
that everybody wanted to help them, not simply to discuss
their failures, and was a proof that he regarded his conver-
sations with the Uptons as confidential. Respect was demonstrated, too, in the planning of interviews. At the outset the
worker set the tone of the contact by writing to arrange an
appointment at a time convenient to the Uptons—a small

courtesy, but important to this family. After this, weekly interviews were arranged for a regular day and time: an appreciation of the importance to the Uptons of knowing that they could depend on his coming then, and a demonstration of his concern in setting aside this hour specially for them. This distinguished his visits, too, from the casual dropping-in which could have implied lack of interest and which could have confused social work with efforts to detect poor home-making. It took time to overcome suspicion in a family who had grown to regard callers at their home as unheralded inspectors of their capability. It was essential to convey a real desire to help, not to criticize, and to give Mr Upton time to learn how a social worker would be used. It was, in fact, almost a year before Mr Upton could make the positive move of asking to be given a training.

It could not be expected that the Upton's life would be all plain sailing after this. The difficulty of learning a new trade in middle life, the reality that the whole family had poor health and that Mr Upton's personality was complicated meant that they would be vulnerable. Mr Upton's adjustment took time and the worker's support was needed through many incidents and uncertainties. But in the period under consideration the upward spiral was started and Mr Upton set on a path towards independence.

Looking back, the social worker realized that in the early stages he had not helped the Uptons as effectively as he might have done. In the first few interviews he had listened to their troubles but had not been sufficiently supportive. In trying to demonstrate a helpful, non-critical approach he had let the Uptons' anger grow to the point that it had to explode. The really helpful thing, however, was that when the explosion came he could show them that he had not been hurt or alienated by it, both by telling them so and by emphasizing that he would be back the next week as usual. Apart from the reassurance of such an experience for the Uptons, this demonstration of tolerance was the beginning for Mr Upton of being more tolerant of himself and of the society he was fighting.

Families like the Uptons come to the social services in great numbers. They are the people who are least helped by their families and friends because they have such difficulty in making and maintaining ordinary friendly relationships; they exhaust people's patience without being helped. They can manage tolerably well so long as the pressures on them are not too great but after a certain point their capacity to cope breaks down. Such families are a challenge to social workers, who often react negatively to this degree of anger and frustration. They, like others, have that wish to help and an intuitive ability to respond appropriately to many forms of need. But it is with people like Mr Upton that goodwill and intuition are not enough. Social workers need to be trained to understand such responses and to tolerate erratic behaviour and even frightening outbursts. It is their job to be able to appraise what is needed so that they know what kind of help to offer to a person in need and how to offer it, and so to play a part also in the effective and economical use of the social services.

CHAPTER V

SOCIAL WORKERS IN ACTION: MR AND MRS BRISTOE

THIS is a record of work by a probation officer with a woman who has been found guilty of stealing. It shows the crisis which may be precipitated for the whole family by this and by the court's sentence. The record has been selected partly because it shows a social worker wrestling with the doubts and setbacks so often encountered on the job and how she makes use of adverse circumstances.

December 15th. I was on duty at West Burnthorpe Magistrates' Court that morning. There was only one woman on the list, Emma Bristoe charged with larceny.

Mrs Bristoe was a small, anxious looking woman in her late forties with greying hair and an expression which reminded me of a baby, bewildered and a little petulant. She pleaded guilty to stealing from her employers, Messrs Higginbottom and Brown, a boy's shirt, valued 15s 11d. She asked to have another offence taken into consideration—stealing from the same firm on various occasions earlier in the month four pairs of silk stockings and a little girl's dress, total value £3 11s 6d. When asked if she had anything to say about these offences she said in a small voice, 'I'm sorry.' She looked like a naughty child. She had three previous offences, one as a juvenile and two as an adult, all of which were for stealing. For the first offence as an adult she was conditionally discharged, and for the second, stealing from a firm where she and her husband were both employed, she was placed on probation for a year. She has not been in trouble since then. The policeman who gave the facts of the case, spoke sympathetically. He said he understood there were marriage difficulties and debts and that Mrs Bristoe had stolen the articles as Christmas presents for her children.

The Chairman of the Magistrates said he took a serious view of this offence and was not disposed to take the matter lightly, but before passing sentence he would like the probation officer to find out a little more about Mrs Bristoe's circumstances. Turning to me he said, "I want to know about the marriage difficulties and the debts.' (From the way he spoke I realized that he had a prison sentence in mind unless there were very good reasons for leniency.)

I saw Mrs Bristoe in a small room at the back of the court. She was very agitated, confused and unco-operative. She said she couldn't possibly stop to talk to me. She had to get back to Pamela. I asked if Pamela was her daughter. She said snappily, 'Yes'. I asked how old she was. 'Six.' I asked if there were any other children. She said there was Tony, aged thirteen, but he had gone to Blackpool for the day with a mate and wouldn't be back till six. I asked about her husband. He worked for a firm of agricultural suppliers and it was his day to go round the outlying farms, so he might not be back until half past seven or eight, though he didn't know she was in court. 'He mustn't know. He wouldn't understand.' Anyway there was no means of getting into touch with him. I asked if the neighbours would help. She said she wasn't on good terms with the neighbours. Pamela would be home for dinner any minute now, so surely I must see she had to get home. When I didn't reply she got angry. 'This is ridiculous,' she said, 'I have been here since ten o'clock, and now it's past twelve. I thought it would be over and done with long ago. What do they want to see me for anyway?'

She seemed unaware that she might go to prison, in spite of what the magistrate had said. I wondered whether she was stupid or whether she was kidding herself.

I said gently that the magistrates were worried because

this was the third time she had got into this kind of trouble and wanted to know why she had done it and how she could be helped not to do it again. To give her an opening I said that I gathered from what the policeman had told the court that she had taken the things for her children. To my surprise she did not jump at this excuse but said curtly, 'No, I took them for myself.' She seemed prepared to leave it at that, but with a little prompting added that she didn't know why she had done it. She hadn't intended to. It was just a sudden impulse. I asked her if she had acted on impulse on the previous occasions. She replied rather sullenly, 'Well, everyone does it, so why shouldn't I?' I said it was very tempting to do this sort of thing when everyone else does it. She said she had been worried lately and was thinking of leaving home. I replied that I understood things had been difficult at home. She said her husband was always finding fault. He didn't understand how difficult it was to manage with prices going up all the time. She liked to have things nice. When she was a child she had been brought up by a stepmother who was always finding fault and punishing her. She never had anything nice, and didn't want her children to go without as she had done. She went on to describe with pleasure various dresses she had bought for Pamela, saying she liked the child to look nice, but her husband was always at her for being extravagant. She knew she wasn't a good manager but she had to have things. His nagging got on her nerves. She suffered from nerves and had been under treatment at Fairfield Clinic. (The neurosis department of our local mental hospital.) She got depressed and had been very depressed lately. She felt the only thing to do was to leave home.

I said it must be difficult to decide what to do. I could understand that she must often want to go away if she was so unhappy, but no doubt she was reluctant to leave her children. She said she thought they would be better off without her. She didn't think they cared for her. She wasn't a good mother, didn't seem able to love them. I said it was difficult to show affection if you hadn't had any yourself as a child. She responded to this by saying, it was true and that really she did love her children although she couldn't show it.

I wondered where she would go if she left home. She said she didn't know. She had no relations. Her mother had died when she was born. Her father had remarried and shortly afterwards had been killed in an accident so she had been brought up by her step-mother who didn't love her. She couldn't make friends, only Margaret. Margaret was like a sister to her. They'd known each other since school days. I asked if Margaret knew about her court appearance. She said she hadn't told her because although she knew Margaret would stand by her whatever she had done. Margaret was the only person in the world who thought well of her so she didn't want her to know. I indicated my understanding of this.

At some point in our talk I asked Mrs Bristoe about her previous offences. She became confused and said she couldn't remember much about them. She said she only committed offences when she was worried, then she couldn't help it. I asked if she had stolen things as a child, adding that many children do if they are unhappy. She did not answer this directly but said that her stepmother used to leave sweets and money lying about to tempt her and then punished her if she took them.

I asked about her husband. She said he wasn't bad really. He was a good provider and never got drunk or knocked her about, only he didn't love her. She hesitated and then said the real trouble was she did not love him. She felt like this ever since Pamela was born. Before that they had been happy together. I asked her if she had a very bad time with Pamela. Yes she had and she dreaded having another child. She thought she was too old now but you could never be sure. I assured her I could understand her anxiety about this and the difficulties it must make in her marriage.

Her husband had been very upset about her last offence, and kept reminding her about it. She felt he didn't trust her and treated her like a child. This made her very unhappy.

Then the neighbours were so unpleasant. It had all been in the papers. She hoped this wouldn't be in the papers. She couldn't go through all that again. It was because of that that she had had to go to Fairfield. She had left the gas tap on and had been found unconscious but she didn't think she had meant to do it really. She had given up treatment at Fairfield because it didn't seem to be doing her any good. I suggested it might help if I had a word with the clinic and she readily gave her consent. I therefore rang the Clinic and they confirmed my impression that Mrs Bristoe was a very inadequate person. She had been treated for mild depression and a half-hearted suicide attempt. They were quite willing to give her a diagnostic interview within the next week, submitting a report to the court. This, it seemed, would be sufficient to enable me to get the case adjourned for enquiry. I very much wanted to visit the husband and estimate the chances of getting the family on its feet again if Mrs Bristoe were placed on probation again.

I did not wish to discuss the intimate details of the marriage in open court so I decided to base my report on the history of neurotic illness intensified by anxiety over debts. I returned to Mrs Bristoe to get details about these. I also thought it only fair to warn her that she might be detained in custody pending further enquiries, which caused a scene. They couldn't keep her. She had to get home to Pamela. Anyway it wasn't fair. She hadn't done anything to deserve it. 'It isn't as if I were a thief,' she said. I told her there was quite a chance she might be allowed to return home during the adjournment; that I would like to know a little more about her debts and financial difficulties so that I could put forward the best case I could for her. We sat down together with paper and pencil to work out her income and expenditure. Her husband's wage was £17 a week counting overtime. He paid £3 17s 6d mortgage on the house. He gave £11 or £12 for housekeeping. Out of this she had to pay £8 10s 0d weekly on her hire purchase commitments. Clearly she could not feed and clothe her family on what remained, even with her own wages added, so the debts began to mount up. They were already owing well over £50, and her husband had told her she wasn't to spend any more, not even on presents for the children. That she wasn't going to have. She couldn't see them go without. She knew she wasn't a good manager but her husband didn't understand.

Back in court I described the financial difficulties briefly. The chairman remarked that £17 was a good wage and they ought not to have got into debt. I mentioned Mrs Bristoe's treatment at Fairfield, remarking that this offence might indicate a return of this illness, and I suggested that the court might wish to adjourn the case for a week in order to obtain a medical report from Dr Foxley at Fairfield. I also mentioned that there was a young child left alone in the house and that the father would not be home until later that night. The chairman after consultation with his colleagues said he thought nothing was to be gained by an adjournment as he had heard all that he wanted to know, then he sentenced Mrs Bristoe to a month's imprisonment and turning to me said, 'You'll see about the child, won't you?'

Throughout the interview I had been experiencing difficulty in sizing up Mrs Bristoe. Her appearance, her offence, her behaviour, her extremely primitive defences all pointed to a woman grown up in years but emotionally still a child. This assessment was consistent with the severe deprivation she had apparently experienced as a child and was further confirmed by the Clinic, so I was inclined to accept it as true, but I still had some doubts. It could be that Mrs Bristoe was a confidence trickster who knew all the answers. She was very much on the defensive, suffered from convenient lapses of memory, became upset if pressed too hard. Previous experience with clinics and with a probation officer might have taught her to make the most of the story of her unhappy childhood, also leaving a child at home in the hope of not being sent to prison is an old trick. Altogether I had some doubts whether she was genuine but if she had been out to make a good case for herself she would have jumped at the ready-made excuse I had offered her when I asked if she had taken the things as Christmas presents for her children. One would have expected her to make the most of this excuse but with curious honesty she had said she took them for herself. I felt she was speaking from her heart when she talked about her badness as a mother and as a wife and that she felt no good to the family. She didn't throw all the blame for her matrimonial difficulties on her husband but took a full share herself. For these reasons I felt she was trying to be honest about herself, and on balance I decided she was probably neurotic and not a fraud but I wanted to check her story with the family and the Clinic before committing myself definitely to a recommendation that she should be put on probation. I think my own doubts must have got across to the magistrates and probably influenced them against making an adjournment. Clearly I had not put my case strongly enough to convince them that this was desirable. I felt bad about this failure because I didn't want Mrs Bristoe to go to prison. I realized this might have a devastating effect upon the family which was quite likely to break up completely under the shock unless I could do something to hold it together.

I saw Mrs Bristoe again, this time under lock and key. She was in a state of despair, crying bitterly and saying that all was over. She could never go home and face the shame of it all. It was useless to try to comfort her until the effects of the shock had worn off. I just let her weep but not for too long, as I had to get something settled about the child before the police car arrived to take her to prison, which might happen at any moment. I let her unload her distress as long as I dared. Then I gently got her round to thinking about Pamela. I suggested I might be able to find her husband through his firm but she couldn't remember the name or address of his employer. There were no friends or neighbours who would help except Margaret. She would take Pamela if I could get her there and she lived in a village, five miles out of West Burnthorpe. Pamela was too young to go by herself. I promised I would collect her and deliver her safely to her Aunt Margaret. I was given instructions how and where to find her. Mrs Bristoe also gave me her latchkey, hire purchase book, family allowance book, £6 in cash and instructions to buy two pounds of sausages from Taylor's, leave 1s 9d on the dresser for the milkman, get vegetables for the family for the week-end and also to tell her husband what had happened and on no account to let Tony and Pamela know she was in prison. I left her looking a little happier after making these arrangements.

I found Pamela and told her that her mother would not be coming back for dinner. She said, 'Oh, I see. She's been kept late at work.' She did not seem at all worried and was pleased at the idea of going to Aunt Margaret especially as it meant a ride in the car. She also enjoyed helping me to carry out her mother's commissions which made her feel important and useful. We found Aunt Margaret, Mrs Cole, at home. She was the mother of a large family and seemed competent, kindly and with an unusual amount of under-standing. She spoke with affection of Mrs Bristoe, saying, 'Oh, why didn't she tell me she was in trouble. She knew I would stand by her.' She spoke as an eyewitness of many of the cruelties Mrs Bristoe had endured as a child at the hands of her sadistic stepmother. This confirmed Mrs Bristoe's story and showed she was not exaggerating. Mrs Cole also spoke of the marriage difficulties, saying that there were faults on both sides. Mr Bristoe was a good husband but he didn't understand his wife, who was very much like a child in many ways. Mrs Cole agreed to let Pamela stay with her children until Mr Bristoe collected her in the evening.

At 6.30 I called at Mrs Bristoe's house where I found Tony and a mate. I told him Mrs Bristoe was quite all right but had asked me to give a message to say that she would not be returning that night. I also gave Tony a note for his father and said I would be returning to see him about eight o'clock. Tony's anxious face worried me but I could not tell him what had happened without his parents' consent.

At 8 p.m. when I returned to the house Mr Bristoe opened the door, his face grey and haggard with shock. He looked older than his wife, perhaps in his early fifties. His face, heavily lined, gave the impression of a man who worried a great deal, and possibly had a bad temper. He led me into the sitting-room and closing the door of the kitchen where Tony was watching TV with his mate, he began questioning me about his wife, showing a great deal of concern for her. What had happened to her? What had she done? Had it upset her very much? Last time she had been so upset she tried to commit suicide. Why hadn't she told him? What could he do to help her? Why had she done it? Whatever she had done he would stand by her. His anxiety poured out in a torrent. He hardly waited for answers to his questions. His distress was so real that I felt there was no doubt about his affection for her, whatever their differences had been. He said he felt he was partly to blame for what had happened. He had not been understanding enough. The trouble was that he was worried to death about their debts. He had a good income and was never out of work but even so there had to be a limit to spending. She couldn't see that. If she wanted something she had to have it, just like a child. He tried to check her and then she took offence. He knew it was his fault. He got irritated sometimes. He couldn't help it. He worried so much he was just a bundle of nerves. It wasn't her fault. It was the fault of the way she had been treated as a child.

Gradually it came out that he had profound feelings of guilt because of the quarrel they had had shortly after Pamela's birth, when he had lost his temper and had struck her. She had never forgiven him and he had never forgiven himself. He tried to make it up but it was no good. If only she'd be a little kind to him sometimes. He came home tired from work. If only she would ask him how he had got on, show some interest, but she never did. She just grumbled till he lost his temper again.

I felt the spate of his grief would never end but at last he calmed down a little and I thought he had reached a stage when I might be able to get him to think constructively about his immediate practical problems so I asked him if he would be able to manage the children while his wife

F

was away. He could manage Tony, but not Pamela, she was too young. When he got my note he had rung up Mrs Cole and asked her to keep Pamela for the night and if possible for longer. She said she must first ask her husband. He was going over to discuss it with them later that evening. He wanted Pamela out of the way until gossip subsided. The children mustn't know what their mother had done or they would lose faith in her. I did not dare to suggest another point of view about this. He kept coming back to the question of what would happen when his wife came out of prison. He was afraid the unkind things the neighbours would say would get her down as it had before. He had clearly been frightened by her attempt to gas herself. We discussed the possibility of a move to another town to get away from the gossip. He kept saying, 'How do I know that she won't steal again? It's the fourth time.' I suggested a return to Fairfield Clinic but he was doubtful, saying it did not seem to have done her much good before. He felt the trouble lay in their anxiety about debts. If only they could get clear of them they might make a new start. I agreed this might help but suggested that they would also need help with their personal problems.

By this time it was 9.30 and I suggested that if he did not get over to Mrs Cole's house soon he would miss the last bus. He was so knocked out by the blow he had received that he seemed dazed and unable to concentrate on the simplest things. I reminded him that if he was leaving Pamela there she would need her night things. He couldn't even concentrate on collecting these. I had to tell him what to fetch as though he were a small child. With Tony's help the task was accomplished and I promised to drop him at the bus stop on my way home. I was worried by Tony's white and anxious face and the knowledge that no one had told him what had happened to his mother but I knew I could not press Mr Bristoe any further that night, and I hoped he would tell the boy in his own time. In any case I promised to come back and see the family after the week-end.

On Monday I rang up the prison welfare officer and explained the situation. She asked me to keep contact with the home and said she would arrange for Mrs Bristoe to see a consultant psychiatrist with a view to future treatment. In the evening I called again on Mr Bristoe. He had recovered from the first effects of the shock and reaction had set in. He was now very angry with his wife for the harm she had done to the family. He said he had decided he couldn't have her back. It was another very long interview in which he again poured out his distress, this time about the children and what the disgrace would mean to them. An account of the case has been in the local papers and the neighbours were beginning to talk. Apparently some unkind things had been said to Tony at school and he had asked his father what had happened to his mother but Mr Bristoe couldn't bring himself to tell him. He wanted to get the children away from the scandal and had decided he had better break up the home and get the children's department to receive Tony and Pamela into care. It was no good trying again he said. His wife had done this three times. There was no reason to suppose she would stop, and he just couldn't go on like this. I said I could understand how desperate he must feel and how hurt by what his wife had done but suggested that it would not really help the children to deprive them of their father as well as their mother. Children can take an awful lot if they have the support of their parents. Pamela was all right for the moment because Aunt Margaret had agreed to keep her and the best way he could help Tony would be to take him into his confidence so that they could share one another's distress and help each other. The thing that hurts children most is the feeling that they are being excluded; I stressed the need Tony must have for his father's support. Mr Bristoe said he didn't know what to do for the best.

We went over all the anxieties and past difficulties which he had discussed in his first interview with me, particularly Mrs Bristoe's irresponsibility with money matters, his fear that she would go on stealing or that she would have another breakdown. This time a lot of anger came out, the accumulated irritation of years which had been submerged under his

love and concern when he first heard the news. I thought the
first reaction was probably the true one. At the present the
chances of reconciliation looked poor but I hoped his basic
affection for his wife would come to the surface in time if
he was allowed to let off steam, though it was by no means
certain that the home would hold together. At the moment
all I could do was to show I understood his feelings and let
him talk. In spite of his anger he showed considerable understanding of his wife's difficulties and the reasons for her
bad behaviour, which he felt was rooted in her unhappy
childhood. He went on to talk at length about his marriage
difficulties and we discussed the different expectations of a
man and a woman in the marriage relationship, the fear of
pregnancy which was perhaps upsetting Mrs Bristoe and the
distress she was experiencing through the difficulty of their
relationship. Then we went back to the subject of the children. I suggested that it would be better for him to tell Tony
what had happened than to let him find out from the neighbours. He agreed but said he couldn't do it. I asked him if he
would like me to do it for him. He jumped at the suggestion.
We both went in to the sitting-room where Tony had been
left on his own. I was at a loss as to know how to begin
this difficult task. I said, 'Tony. You know that your
mum and dad have been short of money and Dad told
Mum not to buy anything else till the debts were paid.'
He nodded. 'Well', I said, 'Mum wanted to get Christmas
presents for you and Pamela and as she hadn't any money
she was tempted and stole some things from the shop where
she works. Now the magistrates have sent her to prison for
a month. That's what happened.' Tony said in an anguished
voice, 'Oh Dad, what will the boys say at school?' Mr Bristoe
said, 'Never mind what they say. Just tell them she's your
mother and you won't have a word said against her.' Tony
said, 'But why did she do it?' I said that although we all
know stealing is wrong the important thing to remember is
that mummy loved them and that she did this wrong thing
because she so badly wanted to give them Christmas presents.
Tony said, 'I would much rather go without Christmas

presents than this.' Mr Bristoe said, 'Whatever she's done she's your mother and you must stand by her Tony. Never mind what people say. We'll stand by this together, son.' I left father and son comforting each other. I was not at all happy about the way I had handled this but I had felt embarrassed and at a loss to know how to tackle it. I was troubled by the boy's distress.

Later in the week I visited Mrs Bristoe in prison. Her feelings had also changed. She now very much wanted to return home, and admitted that if she couldn't do so there would be nothing left for her. She was full of self pity, said that her husband could not love her or he would have written. She seemed quite unaware that her offence and sentence might have caused her family any suffering, or that her husband had any reason to be angry with her. I told her how much concern he had shown for her when I told him the news and how distressing it was for him. I suggested that it might be nice if she wrote saying she was sorry about it and asking him to visit her. She did not rise to the suggestion and said she did not want her husband to see her 'in this place' and she was distressed that the children had been told about her offence. She feared what the neighbours would say. She showed some anxiety about the children and I felt that under all her denials she was anxious to know that her husband had forgiven her. In fact she was too much concerned by the fear of losing their love to be able to put herself in their place. She did not grumble about her treatment in prison. It was the disgrace that worried her. She wanted to go home and start life anew and make amends. She assured me she would never again do anything that might bring her 'to a place like this'. I told her that I thought that if she and her husband were to make a new start they must begin at the bottom by sharing this experience, and I again suggested that she should invite him to visit her. She promised to think about it and tell the welfare officer. A few days later Mr Bristoe came to my office. He said he had decided he couldn't break up his home. He'd married his wife for better for worse—anyway he missed her. Once more he was blaming his troubles on the debts. If only he could get a loan and be rid of the tally-men he thought he could make a fresh start. I suggested that he should visit his wife in prison but he was very doubtful about it. He thought he couldn't take time off from work. The boss was beginning to grumble because he'd stayed away most of the week. He was in such a state of nerves that he couldn't settle to anything and was in danger of losing his job. It seemed to me that he was in rather an hysterical state. I told him sharply that he had better stop running in circles and get back to work. It wouldn't help anybody if he got the sack. He took this advice and the job situation was saved. The following week he got a letter from his wife asking him to visit her in prison. He did so and I heard from the welfare officer that the meeting had gone off well. They had been reconciled to one another and were planning to make a new start when she came home. Mr Bristoe asked me if I would meet his wife the day she was discharged as his boss wouldn't give him the time off. I agreed to do so.

I collected Mrs Bristoe from prison on the morning of her discharge and took her to Mrs Cole's house where she was to spend the day. Pamela gave her mother a great welcome and later came up to her shyly saying, 'I'm sorry I was naughty, Mummy.' It was as if Pamela was trying to take the blame for what her mother had done. Perhaps she just felt that she must have been bad or her mother wouldn't have left her. It was obviously a gesture of affection, which Mrs Bristoe didn't notice. She was too busy talking to Mrs Cole about her own prison experiences. It seemed clear to me that though Mrs Bristoe loved Pamela in her own fashion she had little understanding of her.

I visited Mr and Mrs Bristoe in their home the following week and found the family happily reunited. On my advice Mrs Bristoe had asked her husband to take over the financial side of the household. He was finding it much more difficult to budget than he had thought. Also on my advice, Mr Bristoe was trying to praise his wife for the things she did well instead of blaming her for the things she did badly.

This was making her feel much happier. He'd worked out a plan for coping with their debts by applying to an ex-service association to which he belonged for a loan with which to pay off the tally-men so preventing them from persuading his wife to make fresh purchases. He himself would be responsible for paying off the loan. It seemed a good idea. Tony had been doing a good deal of truanting from school while his mother was away but they hoped he would now settle at school. The neighbours were being much nicer than they anticipated. Altogether they were quite hopeful about the future. I thought this was the moment to break my contact with them. When I suggested this they became very anxious again. Mrs Bristoe had been promised an appointment at Fairfield Clinic in a few weeks' time. I agreed to keep in contact with them until her regular treatment began and that they should come and discuss any difficulties with me if they wanted to. Mr Bristoe came to see me every week for a while, telling me the ups and downs of the family situation and their plans for the future. When Mrs Bristoe's treatment began at the Clinic she and her husband were given regular appointments with the psychiatric social worker and no longer needed to see me. Mr Bristoe's visits to my office gradually ceased, except when he had some special problem which he felt was my concern.

During the next three years I heard from the Bristoes occasionally. They visited me once when Tony was showing difficult behaviour at school and asked my advice. Mrs Bristoe was continuing treatment at Fairfield. Mr Bristoe had ceased to see the social worker but was still worried about his matrimonial difficulties. They visited me again eighteen months later because the matrimonial problem had blown up into a crisis that threatened to break up the home. I paid two or three visits to try to help them to sort out their misunderstandings. I saw them again to say good-bye just before I left the area. Tony had left school and was starting work on a farm. He had caused his parents a good deal of anxiety during his last years at school by his generally disturbed behaviour but it was hoped that he would now settle down as he had always been a keen young farmer and was thrilled with the job. Pamela was doing well at school. Her parents were hoping that she might eventually get into a grammar school. Mr Bristoe had managed to pay off a large part of the debts and his wife was managing to budget much more successfully. The matrimonial friction continued. Mrs Bristoe was still unable to believe that she could be loved and still behaved like a naughty child at times. Mr Bristoe was unable to contain his irritation with her, so there were frequent quarrels. Both had come to the conclusion that this was a state of affairs which was likely to continue. They sometimes felt it was more than they could bear but they also knew they would probably be more unhappy if they were to part.

From the probation officer's account of her work with the Bristoes we know how precariously the family equilibrium had been maintained over the past years. With an unhappy marital relationship, a mounting load of debt and mounting friction arising from it, a breakdown of sorts was almost inevitable. It might have taken the form of one or other partner leaving home, in which case the family problem would probably have come the way of the children's department of the local authority; or there might have been a breakdown in health, as had happened once before, which would have brought them into the orbit of the hospital almoner or the psychiatric social worker; or the Bristoes might have sought help from a family casework agency or a marriage guidance counsellor. Their family problem was one which might have been the proper concern of social workers in many different agencies. It fell to the lot of the probation officer because the breakdown, when it occurred took the form of a criminal offence. But this in itself added a new problem to the old—the problem of society's attitude to crime and punishment and the Bristoes' own feelings about this. The offence, which was the result of an accumulation of social and personal problems, had itself given rise to a whole new crop of difficulties which affected not only the offender herself but everyone connected with her.

The probation officer came into the Bristoes' problem at the point of crisis. They had not asked for her help and to Mrs Bristoe she must have appeared more like an enemy than a friend, since she represented the punishing court and had been sent, it would seem, to pry into her weaknesses before sentence was passed. It was therefore natural that she should want to run away from interrogation and, finding escape impossible, should have been all the more frightened and determined to keep her mouth shut. This reluctance to trust a potential enemy is very different from the initial diffidence of the voluntary client who goes to a social agency seeking help but feels shy when she gets there and has difficulty in stating her problem. Nevertheless the worker's way of dealing with initial anxiety is the same in both cases. She must herself understand it, looking at the situation through the client's eyes and recognizing her need to protect herself from real or imagined danger. Then she will be able to disregard the client's negative behaviour, respecting the client's defences and not trying to break them down too soon. Fear has many disguises—hostility, indifference, denial of the truth, bravado, effusive friendliness, wishful thinking and others—but where there is fear, there is need, and if the worker can recognize this and go out to meet the client with real acceptance and understanding she will be able to overcome the anxiety and gradually build up a relationship.

In an earlier chapter reference was made to the need to listen with understanding of what lies beneath the client's words and actions. This is well illustrated in the initial interview between the probation officer and Mrs Bristoe.

Mrs Bristoe opens the interview by expressing her desire to run away and giving a rational reason for it—she has to get back to Pamela. This is a legitimate concern and the probation officer gives her attention to it, at the same time picking up some useful information about the family. Mrs Bristoe soon comes out with her underlying anxiety—why is she being kept back to talk to the probation officer? She cannot admit to herself that she might be detained in custody but the thought is obviously at the back of her mind. She keeps it at bay by irrational denial and by hostility. The probation officer recognizes these underlying currents but does not comment. She answers Mrs Bristoe's question simply, explaining her role and that of the court in as positive a way as she can. This leads on to the object of her enquiry —the reason for the offence. The client defends herself by blocking, evading and making excuses, she acted on impulse, she says. The probation officer won't let her get away with this. It will be no help to her to hide from the truth so she asks if Mrs Bristoe acted on impulse on all the previous occasions. Reluctantly Mrs Bristoe mutters 'Everyone does it, so why shouldn't I?' This is as near to a confession as she is likely to get and the probation officer immediately responds with understanding of her underlying shame (implied in her tone of voice rather than her words). Throughout Mrs Bristoe has behaved like a naughty child who expects a scolding. When she is not scolded she relaxes and talks more freely. It might be thought that the probation officer is condoning the offence because she does not offer direct cirticism, but it would do no good at this point. Besides there is a world of difference between the client's question which implies 'It can't be wrong if everyone does it,' and the probation officer's answer which implies 'You know it's wrong, but I know how easy it is to be tempted when other people set you a bad example.' Often the words that are spoken are an abbreviation of what is actually being said. Finding her difficulties are understood, the client reveals more and more of her problems, with the probation officer putting in occasional comments to show her interest and understanding. Mrs Bristoe is still frightened but she now sees the probation officer as someone who may be able to help so she wants to confide in her. She may even become too trusting and the probation officer may have to warn her that she will have to tell the court what she is told.

The probation officer has now got a picture of the home background and can begin to make a tentative assessment of the problem. She thinks Mrs Bristoe is probably an immature person who is reacting to her home difficulties in the way she used to act as a child. This kind of behaviour is characteristic of a deprived child, which Mrs Bristoe clearly was, from her account, and it points to a diagnosis of emotional disturbance as the cause of the delinquency. But the probation officer recognizes an alternative possibility, namely that Mrs Bristoe may be a persistent thief who is trying to pull the wool over her eyes. So she is on her guard and decides she must get some external evidence to check her conclusions before presenting them to the court. She decides to ask for an adjournment.

Mrs Bristoe is still pretending to herself that she has nothing to fear, so the probation officer feels she must warn her of the possibility of being detained in custody. This creates a panic and up go the defences. 'They can't keep me.' 'It isn't as if I were a thief.' To reassure her the probation officer tells her, truthfully, that it may not happen, and enlists her help in the preparation of the report, which gives her something positive to do for herself—a good remedy for panic. But in doing this the probation officer may have fallen into the trap of allowing herself to be seen as the 'prisoner's friend' in opposition to the punishing court, a temptation which must always be guarded against. It is all too easy, in any agency, to take the client's side against authority and this does not help. The social worker must always be seen as representing the agency to which she belongs.

Only a tentative assessment can be reached at the end of a short interview. The more experienced and the better trained the social worker the easier she will find it to pick up the right clues and ask the right questions, but the responsibility of making a recommendation about treatment in a situation where the client does not have the right of self determination is very great and should not be undertaken lightly. If the social worker has any doubts she will ask for more time to pursue her enquiries, but she must convince the court that further time is justified and this the probation officer apparently failed to do, because a prison sentence was passed instead. The probation officer had been over-confident that the court would do as she suggested, thus she was taken unawares by the sudden overthrow of her plans. She was also faced with the necessity of rapid emergency action to save the family from breakdown and lessen the distress of the little girl who would be waiting in vain for her mother to return home. The probation officer did not know the name of Mr Bristoe's firm, through which he might be contacted, or the address of the friend, Mrs Cobb. Without these she could do nothing to help so she must get them from Mrs Bristoe before the police car came to take her to prison. This she knew might happen at any moment therefore she was herself under considerable pressure. But Mrs Bristoe was in a state of shock and needed help to express her feelings before she could collect herself sufficiently to think of the needs of her child. When she did so she showed surprising ability to rise above her own misfortune.

This raises another important aspect of casework: timing. The social worker needs to have two time scales in mind, the external one which regulates the length of an enquiry, or the date when a family will be evicted or a patient leave hospital, and the client's own subjective time-scale which measures the moment when he is ready to make a forward move or recognize a truth which has been lurking just under the threshold of consciousness perhaps for months. The client's subjective time cannot be hurried unduly (this is what is meant by 'going at the client's pace') but there is skill in knowing just when to exert a little pressure. Where external time is unlimited the worker can give the client much more freedom to come to the point in his or her own way than is possible where time is strictly limited. In this case the probation officer left the client as long as she dared, having regard to external time, and put pressure on her as soon as she dared to intrude on the client's need to mourn. In pulling her out of her despair in order to meet the needs of her child the probation officer was making heavy demands, but in doing so she gave the client back a sense of her own value as a mother, as a person worthy of being consulted and needed in a partnership to help someone else. The client responded surprisingly well and as she assumed command of the situation the social worker automatically fell into a supporting role ready to carry out instructions and leave the planning as much as possible to the client. This is in accordance with the principle of helping the client to help himself, only taking over when the client cannot cope or is prevented from doing so. In the subsequent interview with Mr Bristoe, who was suffering so severely from shock that he was temporarily quite confused, the worker took command for the time being and told him what to do even about the simplest things like catching his bus and taking Pamela's night clothes with him. This switch from the leading to the supporting role, according to the changing needs of the client, is an important aspect of casework.

The social work process of problem solving is often thought of as taking place in three successive stages: study: diagnosis and treatment. This is a useful over-simplification. In reality all three processes go on side by side and are inter-related. Because treatment takes place through relationship it begins with the first words spoken by the social worker to the client, and because it is impossible for any human being fully to understand another, study goes on as long as the relationship continues. Diagnosis is also continually changing as new aspects of the client's personality or his problem come to light, and this in turn may alter the goals of treatment. Treatment itself is at first tentative. Its success depends on how the client responds, this in turn confirms or changes the diagnosis and modifies the way in which the treatment plan continues. External reality can also upset plans in various disconcerting ways, as happened in this case, and much of the social worker's skill may be expressed in her ability to adapt to unforeseen circumstances within the over-all plan and even to use apparently adverse events constructively.

For instance, the probation officer's initial plan was to

study the family to assess their interrelations with each other, and thus, how they could be helped. She thought of doing this through a remand on bail but when this became impossible she achieved the same result through the client's voluntary request for help, and in fact the way in which each member of the family reacted to the disaster of the prison sentence threw so much light on their character and potentialities that it probably made diagnosis and planning for future treatment easier than it would have been if this had not happened. The probation officer was able to help the family to use their enforced separation as a useful period of stock-taking and a means of bringing them together instead of driving them further apart. This was the form the treatment took.

The work done in this case was essentially short term. It was successful in so far as it prevented the family from breaking under the pressure of the offence and the prison sentence, but it left the basic problem still unsolved. If Mrs Bristoe had been placed on probation it would have been the probation officer's responsibility to help both partners with their marriage difficulties, with or without psychiatric help. In the event, it seemed more appropriate to refer the case wholly to the psychiatric clinic. The probation officer simply laid the foundations for this, giving the family temporary support until their long term treatment could begin. Quite possibly the Bristoes' problems were as such not curable. The family might need support in times of crisis for many years. But given this, they might keep together at least until the children were grown up and able to fend for themselves. This limited goal would be well worth achieving.

No social worker looking back on a case is completely satisfied with what she has done. She sees mistakes and blames herself for missed opportunities. This probation officer no doubt regretted that she had not done more for Tony, the only member of the family to whom she gave no support. She was worried about this at the time but felt that she must not undermine Mr Bristoe in his role as father, because the fact that his children needed him was the only thing that was keeping him going. But was she right about this? Subsequent history shows Tony causing anxiety by his difficult behaviour, which might well be the result of the anxieties and conflicts he endured unaided at the time of his mother's imprisonment. Could the probation officer have found a way of helping him without damaging his father? Or was she in a position when she had to choose between the conflicting needs of two people? If so did she make the right choice?

It is easy to be wise after the event, but social workers are not omnipotent or omniscient and therefore they make mistakes from time to time, and are often faced with situations when they do not know what is the best thing and must just do the best they can.

CHAPTER VI

THE BOUNDARIES OF
SOCIAL WORK

SOCIAL workers are employed in many organizations. Some of them work in voluntary agencies set up specifically to give a service of social casework. The majority, however, work in statutory authorities, either in departments primarily engaged in social work or in social work sections within services established for a different major purpose. Local authority children's departments employ child care officers to work with families where there are problems over the welfare of children within the parental home, or with those needing to be cared for outside their own homes. In the local authority health and welfare departments social workers help the mentally sub-normal and ill, the physically handicapped, the elderly and the homeless. Hospitals and clinics usually regard medical and psychiatric social workers as part of the team treating their patients. Another branch of social work is the probation service which is part of the treatment service for delinquents and those with matrimonial and other problems which may become associated with the courts. People whose social problems arise from the stress of sickness, handicap, family breakdown, bad environmental conditions and material or emotional deprivation or delinquency can thus to an increasing extent become eligible for social work help.

The cases described in the last two chapters, Mr and Mrs Upton and Mr and Mrs Bristoe, could have come to almost any social work agency. It is usually the nature of the symptom or problem at a particular point in time that determines which statutory or voluntary social service is involved, and which others must also be called upon to meet the total need. The function and boundaries of the particular social service will have an important effect on the kind of help social workers can give. They must recognize this and avoid the temptation of hanging on to cases that should be referred to a more appropriate agency or for other professional service. In order that social workers may make the best use of community resources they must be familiar with the services available in the locality. They must also understand the function of related professions so that they may co-operate with them intelligently.

The case of Gordon White shows the interaction of the medical profession and social work. The problem of Gordon's blindness would have been brought to a doctor in the first place, who would have referred him to the specialist service provided by the hospital. The doctors who treated his blindness recognized the social implications of his condition and referred him to the medical social worker. If in the end the doctors decided that there was no hope of saving his sight the medical social worker would refer the case to the welfare officer of the local authority, whose job it is to look after physically handicapped people living in the community. The medical social worker would try to help Gordon to make a successful transfer to the new worker.

Several agencies were involved in the case of Mr Upton. The general practitioner, the hospital, the disablement resettlement officer, a social worker from the industrial rehabilitation unit, a National Assistance Board officer, a health visitor, various charitable organizations and the curate of the local church, all took a hand in helping the family. They gave practical and financial assistance, combined with a great deal of good advice, which only had the effect of making Mr Upton feel more and more inadequate and resentful. He retaliated by playing off one against another, until the health visitor wisely called in the aid of a family casework agency. She realized that it was no good trying to help

G

the family piecemeal: their problems must be dealt with as a whole, and effective treatment should be in the hands of one worker who could co-ordinate the help given by all the others. The worker chosen for this task must come from an agency with a structure that allowed for long-term treatment on a basis of frequent and regular interviews. None of the statutory or voluntary bodies previously involved with the family were so structured.

Unlike Gordon White and Mr Upton, there was no medical problem in the case of Mrs Bristoe. Her difficulties seem to have originated in her sufferings as a child at the hands of her step mother, which had hampered her development to such an extent that she had remained emotionally a child even though she was now middle-aged. This one-sided development is just as crippling to the individual as loss of sight or loss of limb and it may be just as incurable. Her self-centredness, her lack of forethought and responsibility, and her way of punishing the people she was cross with is the behaviour of a child not an adult. The problem of the family was that of having a grown-up child occupying a position of responsibility as wife and mother. In her heart of hearts Mrs Bristoe can never believe she is loved or could be loved and therefore she is unable to give love though she genuinely wants to. She has suffered a psychological disablement which is quite as profound as the physical disablement of Gordon White and Mr Upton and in some ways more of a handicap. The question here is whether the disablement in incurable. Probably it is, if so the client and her family must be helped to adjust to it. The prognosis is not good but there are some positive aspects and therefore there is a chance that with continuing support the family could be held together.

Mrs Bristoe's problems became the concern of the probation officer when the court asked for a report on her home circumstances, and if a probation order had been made this would have been the beginning of long-term treatment, but as there was no order the probation officer's statutory duties ended when she had made her report to the court.

She was able to give voluntary help to see the family through the crisis but then had to decide what would be the most appropriate agency to undertake long-term treatment. She was right in seeking the advice of the psychiatrist who had had Mrs Bristoe as a patient in the past because only a doctor would be qualified to say whether she was suffering from mental illness and whether she was likely to respond to psychiatric treatment. It is right that the patient should be given every chance of help but it does not follow that she will necessarily be able to respond to the help offered: the trouble may prove incurable. If Mrs Bristoe failed to respond to psychiatric treatment it is probable that she would eventually come back to the care of a social worker, either by direct referral or by a recurrence of one or other of her old troubles, which in some ways can be likened to a cry for help. In this event the social worker's task would be to help Mrs Bristoe and her family to make the best of the situation which her personal difficulties make for them all.

Some clients of this type respond better to casework help than to psychiatric treatment. The Bristoes in fact returned to the probation officer later when things went wrong again. The immature, childlike client often responds better to firm but kind treatment than to a completely permissive attitude which makes too high a demand on the client's imperfect self-control. In such a case the social worker is regarded by the client almost like a strict but loving parent who will understand and support all his legitimate aspirations but set limits to his unruly behaviour. It is only within recent years that social workers have begun to understand the importance of this controlling, limit setting function. In the past it was thought that casework was impossible in an authoritarian setting. Now it is acknowledged that in many cases an authoritarian setting is an advantage. It enables the client to regain or gain the security of childhood under the guidance and control of a responsible adult. Many clients are afraid of their own unruly emotions and welcome some measure of control provided it is not excessive and can be seen to be just.

There are advantages and disadvantages in working in an authoritarian setting. This can be seen in the probation service and also in the children's department particularly when children come into care under a fit person order made by a juvenile court. Then the children's officer has to assume the responsibilities of guardianship, if need be up to the age of eighteen and may have to make decisions which are contrary to the wishes of the child and its parents. This calls for skill, firmness and understanding in the social workers concerned. The Children and Young Persons Act, 1963, gives the children's department added responsibility to initiate action in relation to children through taking those who are said to be beyond control to the juvenile court.

Attempting to help with human problems is an exacting and complex task in which no social worker should expect to have all the answers or be expected to carry total responsibility without the support of colleagues. Some organizations provide regular consultation with senior social workers for newly qualified staff to help them to relate what they have learned to the demands of the job and to share in taking difficult decisions; this help is vital if the benefits of training are not to be wasted. Most social workers, whatever their seniority, value the opportunity to consult with colleagues from time to time, either to discuss their handling of specific situations or questions of agency policy. Consultation should be considered a normal part of practice.

Good practice also requires the keeping of adequate records. Each department or organization will lay down its own requirements, while information must also be kept for statistical or statutory purposes. Social workers have an obligation to their employers to keep records in such a way that they work efficiently as members of a team. Administrators must have access to a record which is readily available, clear and up to date, so that they may know what is being done in their departments, both for their own satisfaction and for other official purposes.

Social workers as a whole are in a position to know at first hand how the operation of social legislation and social planning affects individuals and what changes may be indicated by new trends in social need. As employees of social work organizations and as members of their professional associations it is their responsibility to document this knowledge in order to make it available as part of the evidence for decisions about policy changes. It is indeed part of their professional responsibility to share in the movement for social reform, social justice and improvement in the social services.

Social workers also keep records for professional purposes, so that they may have an account of casework with an individual over a period, and can learn from noting trends and changes in a client's needs and attitudes, together with improvement or deterioration in his ability to cope with his difficulties. There is no one correct way of recording. The purpose of the record will indicate the way in which it is kept; it is necessary to be flexible, within pre-determined limits. The three records quoted were selected because they were kept in unusual detail and thus showed clearly the process of work with these three families. They were also selected as illustrations of good practice and of the appropriate use of social workers.

Often appropriate help is not offered at the right time, with the result that situations deteriorate. When this happens more time, more skill and more money are required to try to put things right than if they had been foreseen and dealt with at an early stage. It is true that often no clear-cut cause and effect relationship can be demonstrated between the social worker's intervention and the client's improvement. It may be a combination of circumstances which produces a satisfactory or a negative outcome, and to identify the exact contribution of social work among many other factors is not possible. What can be demonstrated in many clients when they have received help from a social worker is their increased ability to do things for themselves and to take greater responsibility for their own affairs. For instance, Mr Bristoe began to function effectively as head of his family and produced his own plan for getting out of debt; Mrs Bristoe resumed the treatment from which she had lapsed; Mr Upton asked for training which he had been resisting; Mrs White relaxed sufficiently to behave naturally with her adolescent son; Gordon began to find interests and to test himself out in public—the preparation he needed to face a regular job. This is evidence from work with only three families, but social workers in all branches could show similar results.

Caseworkers were for a long time puzzled by the irrational behaviour of many of their clients. Then psycho-analysis began to throw a light on aspects of human behaviour which before had been inexplicable. This new understanding made social work much more effective. A truth has a way of appearing self-evident once it has been grasped and it is difficult for caseworkers now to be certain how much of their present knowledge they would have discovered for themselves without this stimulus. Certainly their debt to psycho-analysis is very great. For a time it tipped casework too far over into psychotherapy, too much attention was paid to the client's development in early childhood, too little to cultural expectations and to the variety of human relations affecting him in the present. Social workers have now recaptured some of their earlier emphasis on the importance of the social environment and are borrowing concepts from the field of sociology, in particular they are now using some aspects of role theory. They now ask such questions as: How successful is this client in his role as breadwinner? In his role as husband? In his role as father? If he is strong in one of these the social worker can strengthen his confidence by recognizing this, which may sometimes also help him to become more able to function in other roles in which he is weak.

The study of society has shown that individual people's behaviour is very largely determined by cultural beliefs and rules of behaviour—what is 'done' or 'not done' in their particular set or neighbourhood group. It is not possible in this book to discuss this important subject in any detail. It must suffice to say that the social elements in the total situation are receiving a new degree of attention. This does not mean that the psychological factors are no longer thought to be important: but social workers need to take both individual personality and social influences upon people into consideration in order to reach a fuller understanding of the problem with which they are confronted.

It has sometimes been suggested that modern casework is the child of a marriage between psychiatry and sociology. If so, like all children, social casework has developed a character of its own which is not identical with that of either of its parents. Psycho-analysis and psychotherapy are primarily concerned with the relationship of the individual to his own inner life. Social psychology and sociology are concerned with group relations and social structure and the ways in which these affect current behaviour.

Caseworkers are concerned with the individual in his social relationships. Their work is centred around stress arising from the demands which are made upon the individual both from without by society, and within from his own nature, with both of which he must somehow come to terms. They frequently work with several members of a family and are therefore concerned with the dynamic factors within the family group—the tensions and interplay of one member of the group with another. Social group work methods are therefore relevant to their work with individuals.

Social workers in Britain have only just begun to think of themselves as members of one profession rather than as medical social workers, child care officers, psychiatric social workers, probation officers, and so forth. Each group is beginning to see how much in their practice and experience they hold in common with social workers in other branches; to consider the possibility of agreeing on a common code of ethics; and to work out an agreed standard for qualified entry into the profession.

We have reached a point where caseworkers can begin to take stock of their heritage and consider what they can truly call their own. They have real understanding of the behaviour of people in situations of stress, and some skill in helping to relieve acute stress. They are beginning to realize that stress can be used constructively to help the client to see the real situation which faces him. They have some understanding of the anxious or angry client's irrational behaviour; and have learned to look below surface behaviour to the feelings which cause it. They are learning to assess when to give support to clients and when to help them to stand on their own feet. They are beginning to learn how to use authority constructively rather than to evade or deny it. They are learning when to respect the client's defences or when it may be possible for him to look, with the case-worker's help, at what he is really doing and so gain more awareness of the nature of his problem and thus more ability to cope with it.

The early social workers, particularly Octavia Hill, sensed many of these things through their own capacity for human relationships. But they could not transmit this to others in the form of either knowledge or skill. Social workers of the present day have identified much more precisely the reasons why this intuition of earlier social workers was often right and why, for example, Octavia Hill's methods succeeded. Nowadays we can train average social workers to help people in ways which earlier were possible only to exceptional individuals. If this knowledge has enabled present day social workers to help more effectively, they can confidently hope that increased knowledge and better skill will enable social workers in the future to help a wider variety of people more surely than is possible at the present day.

The essence of our belief as social workers was summed up by Octavia Hill in the 1860's:

'Alleviation of distress may be systematically arranged by a society; but I am satisfied that, without strong personal influence, no radical cure of those who have fallen low can be effected . . . If we are to place our people in permanently self-supporting positions it will depend on the various courses of action suitable to various people and circumstances, the ground of which can be perceived only by sweet subtle human sympathy, and the power of love. By knowledge of character more is meant than whether a man is a drunkard or a woman dishonest; it means the knowledge of the passions, hopes and history of people, where the temptation will touch them, what is the little scheme they have made of their lives, or would make if they had the encouragement; what training long past phases of their lives may have afforded: how to move, touch, teach them. Our memories and our hopes are more truly factors of our lives than we often remember.'[1]

Annette Garrett, a leading American social worker of this century, writing in 1955, said:

'Casework wisdom includes our original humanitarianism with its warmth and intuitive appreciation of people, our social emphasis, our conscious use of the casework relationship, and added to all these but not substituted for them, a more precise clinical approach. Herein is the ideal of modern casework.'[2]

[1] From 'The Importance of Aiding the Poor without Almsgiving', a paper by Octavia Hill read in 1869 to the Social Science Association, London.

[2] Annette Garrett; 'Modern Casework:—the Contribution of Ego Psychology', in *Ego Psychology & Dynamic Casework* edited Howard J. Parad, Family Service Association of America 1958.

Printed and bound by CPI Group (UK) Ltd, Croydon, CR0 4YY

17/10/2024

01775689-0003